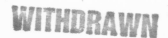

"My Madness Saved Me"

Books by Thomas Szasz

Pain and Pleasure
The Myth of Mental Illness
Law, Liberty, and Psychiatry
Psychiatric Justice
The Ethics of Psychoanalysis
The Manufacture of Madness
Ideology and Insanity
The Age of Madness (ed.)
The Second Sin
Ceremonial Chemistry
Heresies
Karl Kraus and the Soul Doctors
Schizophrenia
Psychiatric Slavery
The Theology of Medicine
The Myth of Psychotherapy
Sex by Prescription
The Therapeutic State
Insanity
The Untamed Tongue
Our Right to Drugs
A Lexicon of Lunacy
Cruel Compassion
The Meaning of Mind
Fatal Freedom
Pharmacracy
Liberation by Oppression
Words to the Wise
Faith in Freedom
"My Madness Saved Me"

"My Madness Saved Me"

The Madness and Marriage of Virginia Woolf

Thomas Szasz

Transaction Publishers
New Brunswick (U.S.A.) and London (U.K.)

Second printing 2006
Copyright © 2006 by Transaction Publishers, New Brunswick, New Jersey.

This book is printed on acid-free paper that meets the American National Standard for Permanence of Paper for Printed Library Materials.

Library of Congress Catalog Number: 2005051419
ISBN: 0-7658-0321-6
Printed in the United States of America

Library of Congress Cataloging-in-Publication Data

Szasz, Thomas Stephen, 1920-
     "My madness saved me" : the madness and marriage of Virginia Woolf / Thomas Szasz.
        p. cm.
     Includes bibliographical references and index.
     ISBN 0-7658-0321-6 (cloth)
        1. Woolf, Virginia, 1882-1941—Psychology. 2. Literature and mental illness—England—History—20th century.   3. Women and literature—England—History—20th century. 4. Woolf, Virginia, 1882-1941—Knowledge—Psychology. 5. Novelists, English—20th century—Biography. 6. Married people—Great Britain—Biography. 7. Woolf, Virginia, 1882-1941—Marriage. 8. Woolf, Leonard, 1880-1969—Marriage. I. Title.

PR6045.O72Z8795   2006
823'.912—dc22   2005051419

The world is there, the world is not awaiting our interpretations but unresisting when we compose them, and it may be that the mere semblance of the world's acquiescence to our metaphor-making leads us deeper and deeper into illusion.

Joyce Carol Oates[1]

Contents

Chronology

1832   Leslie Stephen, prominent Victorian man of letters, born.

1867   Leslie Stephen marries Harriet Marian ("Minny") Thackeray, daughter of William Makepeace Thackeray.

1875   Minny Stephen dies.

1878   Leslie Stephen marries Julia Jackson, widow of Herbert Duckworth.

1879   Vanessa Stephen born.

1880   Julian Thoby Stephen born. Leonard Sidney Woolf, Virginia's future husband, born.

1882   Adeline Virginia Stephen born.

1883   Adrian Leslie Stephen born.

1895   Julia Stephen, Virginia's mother dies, aged forty-nine. Virginia's first "breakdown."

1899   Thoby enters Trinity College, Cambridge. Among his fellow students are Lytton Strachey, Clive Bell, and Leonard Woolf.

1902   Adrian enters Trinity College, Cambridge.

1904   Leslie Stephen dies. Virginia's second "breakdown."

1905   Leonard Woolf appointed to Colonial Service; sails for Ceylon. Thoby starts "Thursday Evenings" at 46 Gordon Square, home of Adrian, Thoby, Vanessa, and Virginia Stephen. Said to be the beginning of the Bloomsbury Group. (The so-called Bloomsbury Group was not a formal organization and who qualifies as a member or belongs to the Group is inherently ambiguous.)

1906   Thoby Stephen dies of typhoid fever.

1907   Vanessa marries Clive Bell.

1909   Lytton Strachey (an overt homosexual) proposes to Virginia, then withdraws his proposal.

1910   Quentin Bell is born.

Dramatis Personae

Bell, Clive (1881-1964). Critic and philosopher of art. Member of the Bloomsbury Group. Husband of Vanessa Stephen Bell.

Bell, Quentin (1910-1996). Art historian, painter, and potter. Son of Vanessa and Clive Bell. Author of a definitive biography of his aunt, Virginia Woolf.

Bell, Vanessa (Stephen) (1879-1961). Painter. Member of the Bloomsbury Group, sister of Virginia.

Case, Janet Elizabeth (1863-1937). Classics teacher and journalist. A highly-educated woman, Virginia's Greek teacher and life-long friend.

Cox, Katherine (Ka) (1887-1934). Close friend of Virginia and of the poet Rupert Brooke. She frequently posed for the renowned painter Duncan Grant in 1912-1913.

Dickinson, Violet (n.d.). Friend of Virginia Woolf. According to Quentin Bell, the first woman Virginia was in love with.

Duckworth, George (1868-1934). British public servant. Son of Herbert Duckworth, a publisher, and Julia Jackson, who, after her husband's death, married Leslie Stephen. Brother of Gerald Duckworth, older halfbrother of Virginia Woolf.

Duckworth, Gerald (1870-1937). British publisher (Gerald Duckworth and Company, Ltd.). Publisher of Virginia Woolf's first novels.

Forster, E. M. (Edward Morgan) (1879-1970). Author and critic. Member of the Bloomsbury Group.

Fry, Roger (1866-1934). Painter and writer. Member of the Bloomsbury Group.

Grant, Duncan (1885-1978). Painter. Member of the Bloomsbury Group.

Keynes, John Maynard (1883-1946). Member of the Bloomsbury Group. Famous economist. Author, *The Economic Consequences of the Peace* (1919), *A Treatise on Money* (1930), and other works.

MacCarthy, Desmond (1877-1952). Journalist and editor. Member of the Bloomsbury Group.

Nicolson, Harold (1886-1968). English diplomat and author. Husband of Vita Sackville-West.

Nicolson, Nigel (1917-2004). Writer, publisher.

Raverat, Gwendolen (1885-1957). Author and leading wood-engraving artist. Daughter of Sir George Darwin, professor of astronomy at Cambridge University and granddaughter of Charles Darwin.

Raverat, Jacques (1885-1925). French painter. Suffers and dies from multiple sclerosis.

Sackville-West, Vita (Victoria Mary) (1892-1962). English poet and novelist. Member of an old aristocratic family. Wife of Harold Nicolson and mother of Nigel Nicolson. Friend and presumed lover of Virginia Woolf.

Smyth, Dame Ethel Mary (1858-1944). Composer, musician. Active, with Emmeline Pankhurst, in the women's suffrage campaign. Composed a rousing anthem, *The March of the Women*, premièred in 1911 and conducted by Smyth herself.

Stephen, Adrian (1883-1948). Brother of Virginia Woolf. Medical psychoanalyst and member of the Bloomsbury Group.

Stephen, Karin Costelloe (1889-1953). Wife of Adrian Stephen. Step-daughter of Bernard Berenson and niece-by-marriage of Bertrand Russell. Medical psychoanalyst and member of the Bloomsbury Group.

Strachey, Alix (Sargent-Florence) (1892-1973). Daughter of famous English muralist-painter Mary Sargent Florence (1857-1954). Wife of James Strachey, close friend of Virginia and Leonard Woolf, member of the Bloomsbury Group. Graduate of Cambridge University, non-medical psychoanalyst, lesbian.

Strachey, Giles Lytton (1880-1932). English biographer and critic. Author, *Eminent Victorians* (1918). Brother of James Strachey.

Strachey, James (1887-1967). English non-medical psychoanalyst. Member of the Bloomsbury Group. Editor and translator of *The Standard Edition of the Collected Psychological Works of Sigmund Freud.*

Wilberforce, Octavia (1888-1963). Pioneer woman physician, general practitioner. Distantly related to Virginia, through abolitionist William Wilberforce.

Woolf, Leonard (1880-1969). Civil servant, writer, publisher. Member of the Bloomsbury Group.

Woolf, Virginia (1882-1941).

Abbreviations

Bell, Q., *Virginia Woolf: A Biography* (2 vols.; New York: Harcourt Brace Jovanovich, 1972). Cited as *Virginia Woolf.*

Freud, S., *The Standard Edition of the Complete Psychological Works of Sigmund Freud*, translated by James Strachey (24 vols.; London: Hogarth Press, 1953-1974.) Cited as *SE.*

Woolf, V., *The Diary of Virginia Woolf, Volumes I-III, 1915-1930*, edited by Anne Olivier Bell (New York: Harcourt Brace Jovanovich, 1977-80). Cited as *Diary.*

Woolf, V., *The Letters of Virginia Woolf*, edited by Nigel Nicolson and Joanne Trautmann (6 vols.; New York: Harcourt Brace Jovanovich, 1975-80). Cited as *Letters.*

Preface

1

The belief that "genius" is a kind of "madness," that "creativity" is neurologically linked to "insanity," and that "insanity" is a bona fide medical illness, a genetic disease of the brain, forms the foundations of the modern secular religion called "psychiatry." Allan W. Snyder, the Peter Karmel Chair of Science and the Mind at the Australian National University and the Anniversary Chair of Science and director of the Centre for the Mind, both at the University of Sydney, states: "Madness, bipolar disorder, schizophrenia or whatever, somehow facilitate creativity.... I wonder if our results with magnetic pulses could help explain why so many geniuses suffer mental disorders."[1]

Virginia Woolf, alleged victim of manic-depressive illness, is an emblem of this pseudomedical fable: She embodies and instantiates the woman writer "touched by fire," a "genius" whose work is at once inspired and thwarted by her "illness." A critic cogently observes: "If you knew female writers from recent trips to the cinema, you might be forgiven for imagining that mental illness came with the job."[2]

This is patently absurd. For millennia, human beings have produced great works of art, no one feeling a need to attribute them to their creators' genius or mental illness. Modern man, however, is satisfied only with "scientific" explanations. Thus, he eagerly embraces the nonsensical pseudoneurological-reductionist view that attributes "creativity" to "genius" or "mental illness," and both to genes. *Credo quia absurdum est.*

Virginia's dramatically crazy behavior, her stature as a prominent feminist writer, and our psychiatrically informed Zeitgeist have led most commentators to take for granted that she was mentally ill. Malcolm Ingram, a Scottish psychiatrist, declares: "Few qualified psychiatrists have commented on her psychiatric history, perhaps

1

because they find little to disagree with in the orthodox view that she suffered from manic-depressive psychosis.... When she wrote at the end of her life that she was going mad 'again,' she spoke the truth and from lengthy experience."[3] This conviction forms an integral part of the vast Woolf literature and mythology. Treated as fact, the claim that Virginia Woolf was mentally ill is adumbrated with endless speculations about the nature of her "illness" and its effect on her marriage and work.[4]

I have long maintained that mental illness is a myth; the term refers to a metaphoric, not a literal, illness. This view is not the product of medical, psychiatric, or neuroscientific research, and cannot be falsified by such research. It is the product of critical thinking and the willingness to reject a powerful, fashionable fiction. The religiously pious person does not doubt that miracles and saints exist: He questions only whether this or that unusual event or unusual person qualifies as a miracle or as a saint. It is the same today with the psychiatrically pious person. He does not doubt that mental illnesses and mad persons exist: He questions only whether this or that unusual behavior or unusual person qualifies as a case of mental illness or as a mentally ill person. The psychiatrically enlightened person *knows* that the medical condition called "madness" exists, just as the religiously enlightened person *knows* that the spiritual condition called "sainthood" exists.[5]

2

We are cast into roles usually before even coming into this world and inexorably after we enter it. We are assigned a name, an age, a gender, and a religion. John Doe, infant, male, Protestant.

Years pass, during which the roles ascribed to us multiply and form our sense of self, the "I." The child says, "I am John, my brother is Michael, my mother is Mom, my father is Dad, and my dog is Puppy." John is being taught his role, his identity. He is beginning to learn "his place" and play his part in his family, school, society, and world.

From an early age, the child is told many other things as well: that he is excitable, or disobedient, or selfish, or clever, or a mama's boy; or perhaps that he is odd and crazy. As he hears such messages habitually directed at him, he is likely to become the person the important others tell him he is. Psychologists call this the self-fulfill-ing prophecy. It is a good term, but it is too narrow. The notion overlooks that the individual cast into a role is not a mannequin whom others are free to dress as they please. He is also an active agent— even as a child, and increasingly as he ages—free (within limits) to submit to and embrace or resist and reject the role-casting.

I regard all so-called models of mental illness—psychiatric, medical, biological, social, antipsychiatric—as fallacious and misleading. Instead, I view all behavior—"mental illness," "psychiatric diagnosis," "mental hospitalization," and "psychiatric treatment"—according to what we might call the Shakespearean or theatrical model.[6] In *As You Like It*, Shakespeare writes:

> All the world's a stage, /And all the men and women merely players: / They have their exits and their entrances; / And one man in his time plays many parts, / His acts being seven ages. At first, the infant, / Mewling and puking in the nurse's arms. / Then the whining school-boy, with his satchel / And shining morning face, creeping like snail / Unwillingly to school. And then the lover, / Sighing like furnace, with a woeful ballad made to his mistress' eyebrow. Then a soldier, / Full of strange oaths and bearded like the pard, / Jealous in honour, sudden and quick in quarrel, / Seeking the bubble reputation / Even in the cannon's mouth. And then the justice, / In fair round belly with good capon lined, / With eyes severe and beard of formal cut, / Full of wise saws and modern instances; / And so he plays his part. The sixth age shifts / Into the lean and slipper'd pantaloon, / With spectacles on nose and pouch on side, / His youthful hose, well saved, a world too wide / For his shrunk shank; and his big manly voice, / Turning again toward childish treble, pipes / And whistles in his sound. Last scene of all, That ends this strange eventful history, / Is second childishness and mere oblivion, Sans teeth, sans eyes, sans taste, sans everything.[7]

Being the member of a community, a nation, a civilization entails joining the cast of a particular national-religious-cultural drama and accepting certain parts of the play as facts, not just props necessary to support the narrative. Thus, we in the West today accept as facts that the earth is spherical, that lead is heavier than water, that malaria, melanoma, and mental illness are diseases. As against this perspective, I maintain that while there are mental patients, or madmen and madwomen, there are no mental illnesses. There is no madness either—in the bodies of the denominated subjects or in nature.

Following Shakespeare and the American philosopher and social psychologist George Herbert Mead (1863-1931), I view mental patienthood as, typically, a role into which a person is cast by his family and society, which he then assumes and plays, or against which he rebels and from which he tries to escape. Occasionally, individuals teach themselves how to be mental patients and assume the role without parental or societal pressure to do so, in order to escape certain unbearably painful situations or the burdens of ordinary life.

In this study, I examine and present Virginia (Stephen) Woolf's life, marriage, work, and psychiatric saga from the point of view I outlined above.

3

When Virginia was a child, she was nicknamed "the Goat." Doctors did not examine her for goatness and no one believed there was "goatness" in her.

When Virginia was thirteen, she was sicknamed "Mad." Doctors examined her for madness and found it *in* her. Virginia and her family and friends believed, and people continue to believe, that there was "madness" in her. A biographer asserts: "The 'Goat', as her siblings called her, had always been 'mad'."[8] Even in death, she is being "tested" for mental illness and found to be "ill." In the modern world, such is the rhetorical power of medical terms, especially terms like "mad" and "insane," which connote the presence, *in* the person so named ("diagnosed"), of a malady with disastrous behavioral, moral, and social-economic consequences.

Unlike mathematical symbols, words are not innocent counters. They are guilty of carrying a heavy load of borrowed meanings, with images and significations associated with their history and uses. The goat is not a particularly attractive animal. It is smelly and stupid. Supposedly, Virginia was called the goat because she was mischievous. So are kittens, but that is not what she was called.

For the rest of her life, Virginia remained fond of pet names referring to animals. She called Leonard "mongoose," and he called her "mandril" (sic), ostentatious nicknames, identifying singularly unattractive creatures. The male mandrill, the largest species of baboon, has a colorful, threatening face. The mongoose, a weasel-like carnivore native to Africa, Asia, and southern Europe, is best known as a skilled killer of snakes. Canada and the United States bar the importation of mongooses because of their destructiveness. Such were the "endearments" Virginia and Leonard exchanged in their private language.

We use the term "endearment" to refer to words expressing affection. I propose to use the term "embitterment" as its antonym, to refer to terms expressing disaffection. The language of madness supplies a conventional idiom of embitterments. Virginia and Leonard often used this language in conversing with one another and with family and friends as well. When Virginia was said to be sane, she couched her disaffection for Leonard in the idiom of snobbish anti-Semitism. Leonard accepted these embitterments as his due. When Virginia was said to be insane, she couched her disaffection for Leonard in the idiom of outrage and rejection. These Leonard did not accept. He, as well as Virginia's family and psychiatrists, repelled these complaints by dismissing them as the symptoms of her mental derangement. (This tactic of dehumanizing the oppressed by dismissing his complaint as a symptom of madness is a characteristic feature not only of modern psychiatry but also of modern politics and, often, of family life as well.)

The language Ernest Jones used in his hagiography of Freud to condemn two of his early critics illustrates this style. He wrote: "[By 1923,] the evil spirit of dissension arose.... It turned out, alas, that only four of us were [loyal to Freud]. Two of the members [of Freud's secret Committee], Rank and Ferenczi, were not able to hold out to the end. Rank in a dramatic fashion presently to be described, and Ferenczi more gradually toward the end of his life, *developed psychotic manifestations that revealed themselves in, among other ways, a turning away from Freud and his doctrines.*"[9] Jones did not simply say that Freud and he felt disappointed in, or betrayed by, Ferenczi. Instead, Jones stigmatized Ferenczi as psychotic. Soviet psychiatrists had good teachers and were good students: They became masters in the art of destroying critics of the communist system as mad, suffering from "sluggish schizophrenia."[10]

4

In 1960, when I first asserted that mental illness is a myth, I meant to remind people that, according to scientific-medical definition, disease is a predicate of *bodies*. Hence, if we accept that definition, we need not examine any particular person to know that he *does not have a mental illness*. My separating literal from metaphorical diseases is a variation on Kant's theme of separating "analytic truths" from "synthetic truths."

We know that bachelors are unmarried without investigating their marital status. The truth of an analytic proposition is contained in the meaning of the words involved. Analytic truths are "truths of reason," based on logic and the precise use of language. Conversely, we know that lead is heavier than water by reference to appropriate observations or reliable records. The truth of a synthetic proposition is contingent on what we call and accept as "facts." Physicians discover diseases, such as malaria. Psychiatrists construct and deconstruct diseases, such as schizophrenia and homosexuality.

Thus, we need linguistic methods to verify or falsify analytic statements, empirical methods to verify or falsify synthetic statements.

Diseases have causes, such as infectious agents or nutritional deficiencies, and often can be prevented or cured by dealing with these causes. *Persons have reasons* for their actions, regardless of whether they are said to have or not have mental diseases. It is as foolish to look for the causes or cures of the behaviors we call "mental illnesses" as it would be to look for the causes and cures of the behaviors we call "religions." Action, behavior, conduct—call it what you will—is goal-directed and meaningful.

Physicians use biological, chemical, and physical *tests* to diagnose disease. Pathologists demonstrate the anatomical and histological *lesions* of diseases. There are no objective medical tests for so-called bipolar illness and pathologists have not found lesions pathognomonic of this alleged disease. The "disease" cannot be objectively "diagnosed" in living persons, much less in persons long dead. How, then, do mental health experts and their acolytes know that a person, such as Virginia Woolf, was mentally ill and that the illness was manic-depression? They know it by *interpreting the subject's behavior as evidence of his mental illness;* in particular, they view the subject's suicide as evidence that his malady is a genetically-determined brain disease/mental illness.

Unsurprisingly, it is mental health professionals and journalists ignorant of genetics who proclaim that manic-depression is a genetic disease, while experts in genetics scoff at the idea. Gordon Edlin, for many years a professor of genetics at the University of California in Berkeley, states: "Just as intelligence came to be seen by many as a genetic trait, so too did alcoholism, schizophrenia, and other behavioral 'diseases' [sic].... The strong emphasis on genes and heredity in disorders such as allergies, sociopathy, suicide, alcoholism, depression, obesity, and others is both scientifically unjustified and ethically questionable."[11] Stanford University bioethicist David Magnus adds: "As reductionism has gained cultural and scientific dominance, the claim that genes are causally relevant is transformed into the claim that genes are of central explanatory importance."[12]

Human action cannot be understood in scientific terms; it can be understood only in *human terms*. In *Asylums*, sociologist Erving Goffman presents a penetrating analysis of madness-and-psychiatry as drama, not disease. Leonard, Virginia, the psychiatrists, and Virginia's family enacted this drama exactly as Goffman describes it:

> Career contingencies occur in conjunction with a second feature of the prepatient's [Goffman's term for the subject prior to commitment] career—the circuit of agents, and agencies—that participate fatefully in the passage from civilian to patient status.... [T]ypically, the next-of-relation will have set the interview up, in the sense of selecting the professional, arranging for time, telling the professional something about the case, and so on. This move effectively tends to establish the next-of-relation as the responsible person to whom pertinent findings can be divulged, while effectively establishing the other as the patient.[13]

All this and more, Woolf biographers, psycho- and neurobiographers, and neurofabulist-geneticists using suicide as a marker for manic-depression ignore. They do so for a good reason. "I am suggesting," wrote Goffman, "that the nature of the patient's nature is redefined so that...the patient becomes the kind of object upon which a psychiatric service can be performed."[14]

The United States is now full of "mental health professionals"—luxuriating in the delights of the *Diagnostic and Statistical Manual of Mental Disorders* (DSM) and the daily "breakthroughs" in neuroscience and neuropharmacology—eager to "deliver" psychiatric services to virtually the entire population. At the same time, increasing numbers of former mental patients reject being cast in the role of patient in need of psychiatric services. Calling themselves "psychiatric survivors," they denounce psychiatrists and psychiatric interventions as harmful, not helpful. Sadly, they tend to ignore their own actions that contributed to their being processed into psychiatric objects, and often make no effort to emancipate themselves from their economic dependence on the role of the mental patient disabled by mental illness.

If we look at human existence free of psychiatric and psychoanalytic "knowledge," we see people's lives as efforts to attain the goals they set themselves (or others set for them, which they accept as their own), and to adapt to the circumstances of their lives. Everyone goes through life coping with his particular problems as best he can and as his circumstances permit.

Why is this seemingly commonsensical proposition so difficult to accept? Because psychiatric fictions have replaced the functions formerly performed by religious fictions. They justify, rationalize, and "explain" many widely shared social beliefs and practices and form an integral part of the civil and criminal laws of modern secular societies. It is in this light that I shall examine the Woolfs' relations to psychiatry and psychoanalysis.

5

Like everyone else, Virginia Woolf had handicaps to overcome. She was a female in a male-dominated family and culture; when she was thirteen, she lost her mother; she was, or believed that she was, sexually abused as a young girl. She also had many advantages in life, or what many people consider to be advantages. She came from a distinguished and financially comfortable family; she was physically healthy and good looking.

Such were the cards fate had dealt her. She played her hand by training herself to be a writer and a mad woman, and she succeeded in becoming a celebrated "mad artist." This is how she saw herself, how others saw her, and how she continues to be seen by people familiar with her life and work. Unperturbed by oxymoronic inconsistency, even the authors who claim that Virginia Woolf was sane maintain that she was "driven insane" by her husband.

Virginia's family, friends, colleagues, and psychiatrists regarded her as having been mad all of her life, a view that, for the most part, she shared. Not surprisingly, a smaller number of authors take the opposite position and proclaim her to be mentally healthy, her "madness" the wellspring of her genius. If we grant that the terms "mental health" and "mental illness" and their synonyms name behaviors, not diseases, and that the terms "creativity" and "genius" are postfacto judgments, masquerading as descriptions and explanations, then we must also grant that these abstract nouns can neither cause nor explain behavior, good or bad.

It is not possible to understand what people call "mental illness" and accept as medical-psychiatric practice as long as we focus on the individual diagnosed as ill, to say nothing of focusing on his brain. Instead, our focus must be on the relationship between the individual considered mentally ill and the persons who treat him as a mental patient. One of my goals in this book is to show, through a study of the life and marriage of Virginia (Stephen) Woolf, that the function of the term "mental illness" resembles the function of a term such as "love," rather than of a term such as "leukemia."

When we say that John loves his wife Mary, we mean that John behaves lovingly toward her. Similarly, when we say that John thinks his wife Mary is mentally ill, we mean that John behaves psychiatrically toward her. If John brings Mary and a psychiatrist together, and the psychiatrist "diagnoses" Mary as mentally ill, then the psychiatrist too behaves psychiatrically toward her. Yet, we often see chronically ailing—"crazy," depressed, hypochondriacal—wives turn into healthy and happy widows after their oppressive husbands die.

William Faulkner understood perfectly that saying that a man is crazy is not at all like saying that he is diabetic, and, more importantly, he understood why it is not the same. Listen to Cash in *As I Lay Dying*: "Sometimes I ain't so sho who's got ere a right to say when a man is crazy and when he ain't. Sometimes I think it ain't none of us pure crazy and ain't none of us pure sane until the balance of us talks him that-a-way. It's like it's ain't so much what a fellow does, but it's the way the majority of folks is looking at him when he does it."[15]

Unlike Faulkner, psychiatrists and psychiatrically (mis)informed biographers and writers interested in the "inner" mental states of an individual deemed to be mad invariably focus on the nature of the subject's alleged illness and its psychiatric management. If the individual is a famous artist, the observers speculate about the correct diagnosis of the illness and its effect on the subject's "creativity." I disdain and reject this approach because its main effect, if not purpose, is that of making the subject less admirable as a person, and less responsible for his behavior as a moral agent.

6

Most people recognize that individuals and institutions—the family, employers, the courts, the state—sometimes use psychiatry as a weapon against the individual: They attribute the role of mental patient to certain persons to control them, if need be by depriving them of property and liberty. But few acknowledge that so-called mental patients often use psychiatry as an excuse for securing special privileges or as a weapon against relatives or the state: They assume the role of mental patient to control others by terrorizing them with suicide, or the role of psychiatric victim to extort money from them.

In the nineteenth century and the early part of the twentieth, it was clear—to psychiatrists and most lay persons as well—that the bare bodkin of madness cuts both ways: that just as psychiatrists may choose to ascribe the mad role to individuals, so individuals may choose to assume that role to avoid onerous duties or, more generally, to escape the burdens of daily decision-making. A hundred years ago, psychiatrists were much concerned with what they regarded as the blurred boundaries between mental illness and malingering, between being mad and pretending to be mad. The incomparable Eugen Bleuler declared: "Schizophrenia cannot easily be distinguished from malingering..."[16] Of course not. All mental illness is malingering (or may said to be a kind of malingering). If it were not, the illness would be called "medical," not "mental."[17]

Even more forcefully, the great German psychiatrist Ernst Kretschmer (1888-1964) declared: "The so-called hysterical person uses his symptoms to accomplish his ends. He puts on an impressive show for us, for he knows that our credulity will free him from an unpleasant situation. He resorts to a *purposeful, studied pretense* and thereby actually achieves his goal."[18] Kretschmer's book on hysteria was first published in 1923. Much has happened since then. At the end of World War I, western European nations were still largely hierarchical societies. The role of power in human relations was undisguised: The rule was, *Quod licet Jovi, non licet bovi* (What is permitted to God, is not permitted to the ox). The psychiatrist "diagnosed" (disease), the patient "malingered" (pretended to be ill).

Today, malingering itself is defined as mental illness. As a result, most contemporary commentators on matters psychiatric suffer from a kind of partial blindness—an existential hemianopsia (blindness in one half of the visual field)—with respect to the uses of madness-and-psychiatry. They can see individuals and institutions using madness-and-psychiatry to control and victimize certain persons. But they cannot see its mirror image, individuals using madness-and-psychiatry to control and victimize certain persons and institutions. This is why everyone who has examined the case of Virginia Woolf has seen and described her either as a victim of mental illness, or as a victim of psychiatry, but none has seen her as a user of madness-and-psychiatry and a victimizer of her husband and others close to her. Hence the legend of Virginia Woolf the mad genius.[19] The abolition of the psychiatric legitimacy of the concept of malingering in post-World War II psychiatry is, as I showed in my earliest writings, a manifestation of this denial.[20]

Our view on malingering has a powerful influence on our interpretation of Virginia Woolf's life, work, and so-called mental illness. Was her alleged manic-depression an unintentional medical illness or an intentional hysterical stratagem? Was it a happening or an action?[21] Kretschmer concluded: "First of all we consider the struggling that culminates in hysterical symptoms simply as *the will of the hysterical person*... Many hysterical mechanisms are closely related to what is commonly called a 'bad habit.'"[22]

Realizing that he was stepping on psychiatric toes, Kretschmer added: "[W]e observe objectively, steering clear of clinical or moral preconceptions and avoiding labels like 'sick' or 'healthy,' 'good' or 'bad,' 'hysteria' or 'simulation';... The question of whether these cases [of 'mental illness'] involve hysteria or simulation will not be considered here."[23] No (conventional) contemporary psychiatrist dares to think, much less write, this way. Doing so would spell the end of his career.

7

The distinction between being sick and acting sick is both an empirical problem and a theoretical problem. As an empirical—medical and social—problem, distinguishing between sick and non-sick persons is a practical task whose efficient performance requires both precise and sophisticated methods for detecting disease and persons skilled in using them. Since empirical determinations are always subject to error, this problem will never be "solved." It can only be *resolved*, with ever increasing accuracy and objectivity.

As a theoretical—epistemological, ethical, philosophical—problem, distinguishing between sick and non-sick persons requires attention to the criteria we use for defining disease and for demarcating it from nondisease.[24] The sick person has, so to speak, the right to act sick; the healthy person does not. The malingerer is an actor, an impersonator, a cheat; his "sickness" is illegitimate. The medical and the moral, the empirical and the epistemological, meet and merge in the difference between malingering and (mental) illness.

Malingering is an action. The person who feigns mental illness plays the role of madman or madwoman.[25] Actions, like ideas, have consequences.[26] One consequence is that the actor may identify with the role and become the role. Another is that others may equate the actor with, and mistake him for, his role, and insist that *he is the role*. Ronald Reagan as "the Gipper" is an interesting and instructive example of both phenomena. Reagan's most memorable role as a movie actor was as "the Gipper," George Gipp, a legendary football hero playing for Notre Dame, coached by the equally legendary Knute Rockne.[27] Reagan became "the Gipper," the player who always manages to score the winning goal.

Virginia Stephen was first cast in the role of "the Goat." Next, she became "the goat who has always been mad." Then she was transformed into the iconic, manic-depressive, female-feminist, genius writer. She was not simply mad, "possessed" by insanity. She possessed "her madness": It was her property, her treasure, her identity. She did not merely snatch victory from the jaws of defeat. She transformed defeat by madness-and-psychiatry into the triumph of literary-psychiatric immortality, a model for future poets and writers—the legendary mad-genius artist.

Madness—if we are willing to look life in the face—is neither particularly difficult to understand nor especially interesting. It seems that way only because we mystify it. The term "madness" refers to a potpourri of emotions and behaviors, expressed verbally or more often nonverbally, composed of a number of ingredients, any one of which may be dominant in any one case. The ingredients are anger, aggression, fear, frustration, confusion, exhaustion, isolation, conceit (megalomania, narcissism, self-dramatization), cowardliness, and difficulty getting along with others.

The proverb teaches that the person who focuses on a tree is likely to miss the forest. Similarly, the writer who focuses on the subject's madness is likely to miss or misunderstand how the person's alleged mental illness fits into the life he has lived and has wanted to live. Psychiatry is, and is expected by society to be, a coercive institution. Psychiatrists regularly victimize persons they call "mental patients" who do not want to be treated as patients. However, psychiatry is, and is expected to be, also an excusing, protecting institution. So-called mental patients often use and take advantage of the exonerations, justifications, and refuges that psychiatrists and their institutions offer.

Contributors to the vast literature on Virginia Woolf's life, work, and marriage fall into two symmetrical groups. Most accept that she was mentally ill as if it were a fact on a par with such facts as that she was English and a woman. A few argue that she was not mentally ill and was misdiagnosed by psychiatrists.

My aim in this study is radically different. I propose to examine how Virginia Woolf, as well as her husband Leonard, used the concept of madness and the profession of psychiatry to manage and manipulate their own and each other's lives.

Virginia Woolf was a victim of neither mental illness, nor psychiatry, nor her husband—three ways she is regularly portrayed. Instead, she was an intelligent and self-assertive person, a moral agent who used mental illness, psychiatry, and her husband to fashion for herself a life of her own choosing. This is not to impute some sort of limitless freedom of the will to her, nor is it to deny that the cultural and social milieu in which she grew up and lived had a profound impact on her and the life choices open to her. It is only to remind us of the primacy of her self as an active, goal-directed, moral agent, responsible equally for her "creativity" and her "craziness."

1

"Whatever we are to call it"

1

Adeline Virginia Stephen was born in 1882, into a distinguished Victorian family. Her paternal great grandfather, James Stephen (1758-1832), a self-made man, was a lawyer, fervent abolitionist, and friend of the famed English abolitionist William Wilberforce (1759-1833), whose sister he married after his first wife's death. He had three sons, all of whom became successful lawyers.

Virginia's paternal grandfather, Sir James Stephen (1789-1859), was a civil servant and one of the great British colonial administrators. Also a committed abolitionist, he drafted the bill (1833) that abolished slavery in the British Empire.[1] He had several "breakdowns," which helped create the belief that the Stephen family was tainted by "hereditary madness."

Virginia's father, Sir Leslie Stephen (1832-1904), a biographer and essayist, was the founder and first editor of the *Dictionary of National Biography*. He attended Eton, was ordained deacon by the archbishop of York in 1855, and became a priest in 1859. However, he lost his faith, or rather, as he said, "discovered that he never had any."[2] In 1864, he declared that he was an agnostic and lost his tutorship at Cambridge. In 1867, Stephen married Harriet Marian, a younger daughter of William Makepeace Thackeray, the novelist. She died in 1875. In 1878, Leslie Stephen married Julia Prinsep Jackson, widow of Herbert Duckworth and the youngest daughter of Dr. John Jackson, a physician, and his wife Maria Pattle (1846-1895), a legendary beauty and published writer. In addition to her two sons whom she brought to the marriage, she had four children by Leslie: Vanessa (1879-1961), Julian Thoby (1880-1906), Adeline Virginia (1882-1941), and Adrian Leslie (1883-1948).

15

2

In 1895, when Virginia was thirteen, she became depressed following the death of her mother. Her family interpreted this perfectly reasonable and understandable behavior as a "symptom" of a (nervous) "breakdown."[3] Tellingly, Quentin Bell, her nephew and biographer, calls it her "'first breakdown' *or whatever we are to call it.*"[4] What Virginia's family and the doctors they consulted called "it" was crucial for determining how they thought about "it," how they related to Virginia, and how Virginia shaped the rest of her life.

Bell continues: "From now on, she knew that she had been mad and might be mad again."[5] Right away, we see how calling Virginia's emotional reaction to her mother's death a "(nervous) breakdown" shaped Bell's understanding of his aunt: To him, it meant that she was mad and destined to always be mad. These interpretations—by Virginia's family when she was thirteen and by Bell when he wrote a biography of her—went a long way toward shaping how subsequent biographers and commentators analyzed and explained Virginia's life. Obviously, Virginia could not have "known" that "she had been mad and might be mad again." She was told that she was mad, others defined her as "mad." No one at age thirteen has the information or power necessary to rebut such a "diagnosis," to reject the mad role. Tragically, she never made a serious attempt to do so. On the contrary, she embraced the role and made playing it an integral part of her life strategy—to her profit as well as her peril.

Virginia was perfectly well until her father died in 1904. The four grown Stephen children—Vanessa, Thoby, Virginia, and Adrian— were now freed of parental control. Before assuming their new, independent lives, they went traveling in Europe. On the Continent, Virginia had "tantrums." After returning home, she jumped from a window so close to the ground that the leap caused no physical injury. Bell's verdict was: "All that summer she was mad,"[6] reprising his earlier obtuse interpretation of Virginia's mourning a beloved parent as a mental illness, and omitting that, unlike her siblings, Virginia was very close to her father. She loved him dearly: He was her teacher and companion, and she was his favorite child.[7]

Bell's account of the Stephen sisters' differing reactions to their father's death reflects the different ways we tend to view happy and unhappy behavior. He presents Vanessa's happiness at becoming an independent adult as *motivated* by her relief at becoming her own master. In contrast, he presents Virginia's unhappiness at finding herself free but unprepared for independence as *caused* by her mental illness. The role-casting is complete, once and for all: Vanessa is sane, Virginia, insane.

Virginia had good reasons to feel depressed and despairing. While she had inherited money from her father sufficient to live on, she was not wealthy enough to be considered an heiress. Educated at home, she had no formal schooling. In any event, earning a living was not a serious option for a young woman of her class. Unemployable, sexually and temperamentally disinclined to marry, and well on her way to being defined as crazy by her family and friends, Virginia viewed her future as a void she had no idea how to fill. The death of her father liberated her from parental controls, but she was woefully unprepared to make use of her freedom. Chronologically, legally, and physically, she was an adult, a beautiful, young woman, member of a distinguished, upper-class English family. Existentially, she was an uneducated, unhappy, confused adolescent. What was she to do with her life? She was familiar with the life of the literary person, her father, and decided to embark on the voyage of such a life. She spent the next eight years preparing herself to become a writer. Her leap from a window in 1904 was not a suicide attempt. In 1904, Virginia was an intelligent, twenty-two-year-old woman. She knew how people who want to die kill themselves, for example, by jumping from a high building or ingesting an overdose of sleeping pills. She did not want to die. She wanted to live, but needed a break, time-out to grow up and prepare herself for a meaningful life.

Virginia's siblings were better prepared to deal with their liberation from a domineering father. Thoby, educated at Cambridge, did not have to face the problem of becoming an independent adult: He died of typhoid fever, aged twenty-four, not long after his father's death. Adrian, also educated at Cambridge, became a physician, trained as a psychoanalyst, and married a fellow physician and psychoanalyst. Vanessa attended art school, married, had children and lovers, and became a recognized painter: "[She] had got what she wanted—her freedom," writes Bell. "Her happiness in being delivered from the care and the ill-temper of her father was shockingly evident."[8]

Virginia's family and friends belonged to the privileged class. Highly educated—some became psychoanalysts—they could have attuned themselves to her needs. But they were unable or unwilling to put themselves in her shoes. They failed to see her as a young woman faced with an empty and useless life, terrified by the challenges of sex and adulthood. They chose to misinterpret the non-verbal dramatization of her dilemma and despair as evidence of the recurrence of a medical malady, madness, from which she was doomed to suffer the rest of her life. Henceforth, Virginia's leap from a low window was transformed into a legendary bona fide suicide attempt and transmitted from family member to family member, friend to friend, learned article and book to more learned articles and more books. Who could ever doubt that she was mad? She bore the classic stigmata of insanity: melancholia and attempted self-murder.

Eight years pass. In 1912, Virginia was thirty years old, on the brink of becoming an "old maid." If she expected to marry, she could not wait much longer. She was eager to escape the status of spinsterhood. At the same time, she felt repelled by heterosexual, or indeed any, intimacy. Nor was she willing to submit to a husband in a traditional, male-dominated marriage. This precluded marriage to a man above her social rank or superior to her in accomplishment. Marrying Leonard Woolf—whose Jewishness she despised and whom she could dominate with her madness and genius—solved the problem of spinsterhood, and created a host of new problems.

3

Leonard Woolf, the son of a successful Jewish barrister, was educated at Cambridge, and had a promising career in the Civil Service. His deepest desire was to shed his Jewish identity and be accepted as an English socialist intellectual and man of letters. A devout Fabian and snob, he loved money and the comforts it could buy.

At Cambridge, Leonard met John Maynard Keynes, Lytton and James Strachey, and Thoby Stephen. He became a member of the Apostles and of a small band that was to form the Bloomsbury group. Other famous members of this group were the poet Rupert Brooke, the painter Duncan Grant, the author Edward Morgan Forster, the journalist Desmond MacCarthy, and the author Gwendolen Raverat.

It was through Thoby that he met the Stephen sisters. Virginia's first impression of Leonard rested on a report by Thoby: "And then Thoby...would switch off to tell me about another astonishing fellow—a man who trembled perpetually all over... He was a Jew. When I asked why he trembled, Thoby somehow made me feel that it was part of his nature—he was so violent, so savage; he so despised the whole human race."[9] This is an uncannily accurate mini-portrait of Leonard Woolf, a man so consumed with hatred that his whole body trembled. Often his hands shook so violently that he was unable to sign his name. One night, in a sort of somnambulistic fury, he dislocated his thumb. He told Thoby that he "dreamt he was throttling a man and dreamt with such violence that when he woke up he had pulled his own thumb out of joint."[10] This was the man who viewed himself as a dedicated social reformer, the benefactor of mankind, and lifelong nurse to a "sick" wife. I shall say more about Leonard later. Here it is enough to mention that, during World War I, he was rejected from military service as mentally unfit, a deferment then granted very rarely.

Leonard was eager to marry one of the Stephen sisters. His first choice was Vanessa, who was not interested in him. He settled for Virginia. Before consenting to marrying Leonard, she wrote him a remarkable letter, warning him of the difficulties that would await them. Yet, she expressed her willingness to take him as her husband. The letter is a fearfully forthright document, articulating every one of the problems destined to cause them misery.

On May 1, 1912, Virginia wrote: "It seems to me that I am giving you a great deal of pain...and therefore I ought to be as plain with you as I can..."[11] The theme of Virginia's "giving pain" to Leonard recurs throughout the marriage and the words, "I am giving you a great deal of pain" are repeated, almost verbatim, twenty-nine years later in the suicide note she leaves him. This has not prevented writers from viewing Virginia as Leonard's helpless victim, the weak and helpless wife tyrannized and abused by the domineering-misogynist husband.

Virginia's letter begins by her remarking that, if they married, Leonard would have to give up his promising career with the Colonial Service. For seven hard years, Leonard had served the Empire, which he loathed, and risen to a high position, ruling the Ceylonese (now Sri Lankans). Virginia's joining him in a conventional marriage—giving up her cosseted life in London for that of the wife of a high-raking Colonial officer in some far off place in the Empire—was obviously not an option.

Next, Virginia bracketed Leonard's lust and Jewishness, both of which she experienced as alien, alienating, and abhorrent: "I feel angry sometimes at the strength of your desire. Possibly your being

Jewish comes in also at this point. You seem so foreign.... As I told you brutally the other day, I feel no physical attraction in you. There are moments—when you kissed me the other day was one—when I feel no more than a rock."[12]

Even her nephew and loyal hagiographer, Bell, acknowledges that Virginia was put off by Leonard's Jewishness, a feeling she must have acquired as effortlessly as she acquired the accent of her class. Virginia felt repelled by Leonard, both as a person and as a potential lover. It is important to note that, in this letter, Virginia articulated many of the conflicts that the couple were no longer willing to acknowledge after they married.

From this moment on, the "sane" Virginia averted her eyes from the bitter truths of her marriage. She denied that she was, literally, *mad (angry) at* Leonard. At the same time, during her "breakdowns," Virginia displayed "symptoms" that expressed precisely this painful reality. In turn, those around her defined these communications as the delusions of her sick mind; after she "recovered," Virginia agreed with this face- and marriage-saving interpretation; and, after Virginia died, virtually all contributors to the vast Woolf literature bought this fable.

On August 10, 1912, Virginia Stephen and Leonard Woolf were married at St. Pancras Registry Office. They had many reasons to marry, but loving each other was not one of them. Nor was having sex or children. Virginia wanted to occupy the social role of a married woman. She aspired to what American women in the postwar years often called the "MRS. degree." Leonard, too, was eager to wed and willing to marry her on whatever terms she set. She married down, taking as her husband an odd outsider, a Jew with no personal distinction or family wealth, an ordinary man who had to work for a living or depend on his wife's money. He married up, taking as his wife a "mad" member of the English intellectual and social elite, a woman repelled by Jews and male sexuality.

Admittedly, Virginia was an odd person, and she knew it. The epitome of what men used to call a "frigid woman," she had odd habits of dressing and eating. She was frigid not only sexually but also existentially: She was determined to protect herself from being "known," carnally or spiritually. Yet, she wanted to marry. Thus, she chose to marry a man who was not only culturally alien and socially inferior to her, but who was so consumed with his own conflicts, confusions, and prejudices that he was neither interested in or capable of understanding her, or anyone else for that matter. Keynes biographer Roy Harrod offers this pertinent observation about Leonard's personality: "When I told him [Leonard Woolf] that I could not regard [G. E.] Moore's philosophy (as distinct from his personality) with respect, he seemed deeply offended and began to take up the attitude of a headmaster. I felt I was in serious danger of corporal punishment.... Unfortunately, I knew a great deal more about philosophy than Woolf; his defense was quite trivial. I hastily changed the subject."[13]

Leonard's autocratic, self-centered personality made him an ideal husband for Virginia. She could shut him out of her life—genitally, verbally, spiritually—and he would accept it uncomplainingly. That was his side of the bargain, his just desert for wanting to marry a gentile, English, upper-class, frigid, madwoman.

Leonard, in turn, rationalized his wife's contempt for and hatred of him by invalidating the transparent meaning of her behavior as the meaningless symptoms of madness. "Writers," remarked W. H. Auden, "can be guilty of every kind of human conceit but one, the conceit of the social worker: 'We are all here on earth to help others; what on earth the others are here for, I don't know.'"[14] Although Leonard regarded himself as a writer, at heart he was a social worker: He knew that Virginia was "sick" and "needed help"—*his* help.

4

Like all married couples, Virginia and Leonard had to face the issues of sex and children. They quickly arrived at a compromise. She denied him sex, which he wanted, or told himself he did, but she did not want. He denied her children, which she wanted, or at least told herself she wanted, but he did not want. They and their friends interpreted their relationship—based largely on mutual deception and self-deception—as a perfect "marriage of true minds."[15]

We know that Virginia came to regret not having children. We don't know if Leonard regretted not having sex with Virginia. Nor do we know whether he had extramarital sexual relations. All we know about his sex life is that during his service to the Empire, he was sexually active with young Ceylonese women over whom he exercised God-like powers, and that he felt soiled by the experience.

While Virginia treated conjugal intercourse as if it were rape and refused to submit to Leonard sexually, she treated psychiatric rape by Leonard and his deputies as if it were medical treatment and sub-mitted to it. This unspoken contract constituted the strongest bond between them. After almost thirty years of this charade, having long ago rejected divorce and personal independence as existential op-tions, Virginia's only way out of the marriage was suicide.

Naively, Bell observes: "Even before her marriage, they must have suspected that Virginia would not be physically responsive, but prob-ably they hoped that Leonard, whose passionate nature was never in question, could effect a change... It is proof of their deep and un-varying affection that it was not dependent upon the intense joys of physical love."[16] Bell is denying evidence that he himself cites in the very next paragraph. While on her honeymoon, Virginia wrote her old friend, Ka (Katherine) Cox: "Except for a sustained good humor (Leonard shan't see this) due to the fact that every twinge of anger is at once visited upon my husband, I might still be Miss S."[17] Virginia did not explain why she was angry at Leonard. She contin-ued to be angry at him throughout her life. Virginia and Leonard, both full of anger, were typical "bleeding-heart" socialists whose character Edmund Burke (alluding to Rousseau) satirized thus: "Be-nevolence to the whole species, and want of feeling for every indi-vidual with whom the professors come in contact, form the charac-ter of the new philosophy."[18] In their hearts, Virginia and Leonard were full of love for mankind in the abstract; in their day-to-day behavior, they were domineering, nasty, and snobbish toward indi-viduals, especially their social inferiors.

Virginia's attitude toward sex was an open secret in Bloomsbury. Vanessa consoled Leonard, telling him that she thought "she [Vir-ginia] never had understood or sympathized with sexual passion in men."[19] Vita Sackville-West observed: "She [Virginia] dislikes the possessiveness and love of domination in men. In fact, she dislikes the quality of masculinity."[20]

Virginia realized that, as a wife, she had a marital obligation to have sex with her husband. However, the Bloomsburians were as notorious for disdaining their duties to family and friends as they were for demanding their rights to fulfill their desires, regardless of promises or social conventions. Though a founding member of the Bloomsbury group, this characterization does not fit Leonard. In more ways than one, he was deviant, an outsider: He was Jewish, heterosexual, and dutiful. Virginia fit the Bloomsbury ideal much better.

During the first months of the Woolf marriage, the issue of pro-creation appeared to have been left in limbo. At the end of 1912, Virginia, according to Bell, "was still cheerfully expecting to have children."[21] Leonard was waiting to disabuse her of that notion, once and for all: "Leonard already had his misgivings, but I do not think that Virginia became aware of them until the beginning of 1913."[22] This, I think, is putting the matter too mildly, indeed distorting it. The evidence is clear that Leonard never wanted to have children. Instead of admitting it, he attributed *his decision not to have children* to Virginia's madness. To realize this plot, he needed the coop-eration of physicians.

In January 1913, Leonard went mad-doctor shopping, looking for a physician who would agree with him that he had married a madwoman, unfit for motherhood. First, he raised the issue with Dr. George Savage, a prominent physician and alienist, who had known the Stephen family and Virginia since she was a child." Savage, "in his breezy way, had exclaimed that it [having children] would do her a world of good."[23] This was not what Leonard wanted to hear. He then consulted Maurice Craig,[24] Theophilus B. Hyslop,[25] and Jean Thomas, who kept a nursing home and knew Virginia well. "Their views differed but in the end Leonard decided and persuaded Virginia to agree that, *although they both wanted children*, it would be too dangerous for her to have them."[26] Virginia and Leonard were masters at deception and self-deception. Famously, Polonius enjoins Hamlet: "This above all things: to thine own self be true." Virginia and Leonard made a virtue of being untrue to themselves. Ostensi-bly, Virginia agreed with Leonard that she ought to forgo mother-hood as it posed too great a risk for her mental well being. Whether this was true or false is not the sort of thing about which a distant observer could render a meaningful opinion. However, as with any decision, especially a "medical" decision, one must weigh the risks of doing X against the risks of not doing X. There is no evidence that Virginia or Leonard had done so. That was a big mistake. Virginia's remaining childless was not free of risk.

For many women, having children is essential for personal fulfill-ment, and I dare say for many men as well. In traditional cultures, motherhood is a woman's primary social role and source of mean-ing and purpose in life. To various degrees, this remains true in modern societies as well. It was still true in Virginia's day. It is also important to note that, in Virginia's social milieu, mothers did not raise their children. Nurses, governesses, tutors, and boarding schools did that. Bell recognized that the decision to remain childless "was to be a permanent sense of grief to her and, in later years, she could never think of Vanessa's fruitful state without misery and envy."[27]

This is not surprising. When she married, Virginia was not driven by career aspirations, which might have mitigated the intensity of her *need to love*. I use the phrase, "need to love," advisedly, as I believe it is a need similar to the need for food and sex. This need is normally gratified by loving *one's own* spouse, children, and sexual partners. We love our children not only because we know they need loving, but also because we have a need to love that we satisfy by loving them.[28] The fundamental biological basis of loving and its close connection to eating is revealed in the saying, "I love you so much I could eat you up." (There are similar sayings in German, French, Spanish, and Hungarian, and perhaps in other languages.)

To be sure, Virginia was notably deficient in all three needs. She was anorectic, unerotic, and unloving. Nevertheless, in some measure, she experienced the need to eat, have sex, and love, and she might have become a better, more fulfilled and complete person had she had and loved a child. Savage might well have been right—motherhood might have been good for Virginia. It might have given her someone to love and hence the kind of stability she so badly needed. However, Leonard wanted to be the stabilizer, and he got his wish.

5

Ostensibly, Leonard wanted to protect Virginia from what he regarded as the psychiatric perils of motherhood. In fact, because he did not want to be a father, he schemed to justify his depriving her of bearing children. Virginia correctly perceived that Leonard did not want to have children and was determined to deny her the opportunity to have any. She complied, but not without a sadomasochistic protest. Instead of resting their marriage on their mutual obligations to one another and their children, Virginia and Leonard rested it on her career as a madwoman and his career as her caretaker.

A few months after a "sexually unsuccessful" honeymoon, Leonard proceeded to psychiatrically deceive and incriminate Virginia: He schemed to find a mad-doctor willing to declare her mad, mentally unfit to have children. Savage, as we have seen, refused to play the part Leonard had assigned him. Leonard sought a second opinion, more to his liking. In his autobiography, he naively wrote: "It was to [Sir Henry] Head that I wanted her to go, but I had always anticipated insuperable difficulties to getting her agreement to consult him. *She could not possibly have known that I had consulted him*, and, had she known, in her then state of mind, it would naturally have influenced her against him."[29] In other words, behind Virginia's back, Leonard consulted Head, told him that Virginia was crazy and ought not to have children, and turned to Head solely for a professional validation of his decision.

"[W]e went to see Head in the afternoon," Leonard continues. "I gave my account of what had happened and Virginia gave hers. He told her that she was completely mistaken about her condition; she was ill, *ill like a person who had a cold or typhoid fever*; but if she took his advice and did what he prescribed, her symptom would go and she would be quite well again, able to think and write and read; she must go to a nursing home and *stay in bed for a few weeks, resting and eating*."[30]

Virginia now had the recommendation of two mental health experts, one of whom advised her to have children, the other not.[31] The second also declared her to be in need of immediate psychiatric treatment in a private madhouse, euphemistically called a "nursing home." The opinions of both doctors were just that: opinions. Virginia was free, de facto as well as de jure, to reject Head's recommendation. To be sure, Leonard could have tried to commit her. Virginia should have realized that Leonard was too eager to have her defined as mad and to delegate her "management" to psychiatric personnel. However, that would have required her to face the facts, cut her losses, leave Leonard, and have the marriage annulled. Such a decisive course of action was contrary to her nature; also, it would have entailed serious loss of face.

Leonard succeeded in trapping Virginia, at least for the moment. She then did what people who feel trapped often do: She tried to kill herself or, perhaps more likely, made a dramatic "suicide attempt." Leonard offered the following account of the hours following their visit to Head: "We returned to Brunswick Square and then catastrophe happened. Vanessa came and talked to Virginia, who seemed to become more cheerful. Savage had not known that we were seeing Head and a rather awkward situation had arisen about that."[32]

Leonard had violated medical etiquette. Wanting to set the record straight, Head asked Leonard to go see Savage and explain "how it had come about that I had brought Virginia to see him." He went off to do that, leaving Virginia in the company of Ka Cox. He had barely arrived at Savage's office when he received a desperate telephone call from Ka, informing him that Virginia had fallen into a deep sleep. "I hurried back to Brunswick Square and found that Virginia was lying on her bed breathing heavily and unconscious. She had taken the Veronal tablets from my box and swallowed a very large dose. I telephoned Head and he came, bringing a nurse."[33]

We are not told why Leonard had in his possession a large quantity of barbiturates, presumably prescribed for Virginia. In any case, he was evidently carrying this around on his person, in a bag, which he had left unguarded, and, unbeknown to Ka Cox, in Virginia's bedroom. It is tempting to speculate that Leonard had set up his wife to make a suicide attempt and thus seal her fate as a mental patient requiring psychiatric care.

Not surprisingly, Virginia's taking an overdose of Veronal was quickly discovered—that's why Ka Cox was there. Her stomach was washed out and, physically, she was none the worse for it. Psychiatrically, she was destroyed: Her act was categorized as a "serious suicide attempt," a pathognomonic symptom of serious mental illness. For months, she remained "severely disturbed"—demanding, for example, that Leonard stay away from her—and was cared for by nurses around the clock. Ingram describes this period: "From the Spring of 1914 she was slowly convalescing, typing as a form of occupational therapy, her writing and reading still strictly rationed. By the time war was declared in August she was well...by mid-September she was in excellent health."[34]

Irrevocably typecast as a madwoman, she played that role for the rest of her life, and beyond the grave. That was and is the psychiatric, and hence the "factual," account of Virginia Woolf's 1913 suicide attempt and its aftermath. In my view, her taking an overdose of sleeping pills, "accidentally," made readily available to her by Leonard, was her nonverbal response to being psychiatrically raped and denied motherhood. I interpret her "recovery" as her becoming tired of being sidelined from life. She became more docile, at least for a time. Her breakdown was her decision, a retaliation against Leonard for taking her to see Head, and her recovery was her decision, bringing down the curtain after the drama had served its purpose. She turned her madness on and off the same way for the rest of her life.

In his autobiography, Leonard provides a detailed account of Virginia's 1913 suicide attempt, at the end of which he adds: "I do not know what the present state of knowledge with regard to nervous and mental diseases is in the year 1963; in 1913 it was desperately meager."[35] This is a disingenuous and crassly self-serving remark. The fact is that Leonard used madness and psychiatry like an expert: He used it to deny and cover up the phoniness of his marriage, to control Virginia, and to avoid military service in World War I.

When a woman displays dramatic despair shortly after delivering a baby, psychiatrists say she suffers from postpartum psychosis. I say she suffers from the realization of having made an irreversible, life-altering decision, a choice that, in retrospect, she regrets, and one having consequences with which she feels unable to cope. *Mutatis mutandis*, Virginia suffered from "postmarital psychosis," the realization of having made an irreversible, life-altering decision, a choice that, in retrospect, she regretted and with which she felt unable to cope. It dawned on her that she had acquired a husband she did not want but lacked the strength to leave.

The Woolfs' marital predicament was resolved by their having Virginia play the roles of mental invalid and literary genius, and Leonard play the roles of mental nurse and literary impresario of his mad-genius wife. "Each day, Leonard noted down his wife's mental state: Fairly well, fair night, good night, fairly good night."[36] Throughout their marriage, Leonard kept a log of Virginia's mental state, the "nursing notes" of a "nursing" husband.

2

"In the head you know"

1

Our initial identity, like our very being, is determined and defined by our parents, and, derivatively, by the language and society into which we are born. Parents identify us by giving us "proper" names. There is wisdom in the Roman adage, *Nomen est omen.* From an early age, parents classify their offspring as easy or difficult babies, obedient or rebellious children, and so forth. With maturity, we acquire the ability and power—within certain limits set by biology, family, society—to define ourselves, in opposition, if need be, to identifications imposed on us by others.

The Stephen family, as we have seen, defined Virginia as mentally ill when she was barely thirteen, and clung to that identification throughout her life as well as after her death. How did Virginia respond to being labeled mentally ill? Did she view herself as sane or insane? Did she reject and rebel against the role of mental patient, or did she accept and embrace it? Did she try to understand what mental illness *is*? Instead of asking such questions, Woolf students assume that Virginia had no part in being identified as mad. This is not true. She played an important role in being identified as a mental patient and she deliberately exploited that role for her own purposes.

The practice of individuals labeling troublesome relatives—especially husbands stigmatizing their wives—as insane, and incarcerating them in madhouses, was common long before Virginia Stephen was born.[1] *Pari passu*, the victims—especially the betrayed wives—frequently became newsworthy for rejecting and rebelling against being identified and imprisoned as mad.[2] Brief mention of the mental hospitalization of two famous women, whose situation had much in common with Virginia's, is in order here.

Rosina (Wheeler) Bulwer Lytton (1802-1882) was a famous Irish beauty, a prematurely feminist writer, and the wife of Sir Edward Bulwer Lytton (1803-1873), Member of Parliament and celebrated Victorian novelist. Their marriage was short-lived. After producing two children, the couple separated in 1836 and spent the next forty years annoying each other.[3] Intending to injure her husband's political aspirations, Rosina embarrassed him publicly. "He retaliated by having her certified insane, employing the same doctor who had certified the wives of Dickens and Thackeray."[4] Unlike Virginia, Rosina rejected the role of madwoman imposed on her, "insisting through the newspapers that she was sane and, therefore, had been wrongly incarcerated. She gained her freedom in just over three weeks."[5] In her memoir, *A Blighted Life*, she had the last word.[6]

To contemporary readers, especially feminists, Charlotte Perkins Gilman (1860-1935), the author of *The Yellow Wallpaper* (1892), is a more familiar name.[7] Gilman, an upper-class, intelligent New Englander and niece of Harriet Beecher Stowe, became "nervous" after the birth of her child and was declared to be suffering from "hysteria." She was treated with S. Weir Mitchell's famous "rest cure," which consisted of bed rest, complete mental and physical inactivity, coerced feeding, and isolation from family and friends. After a month of that "treatment," Gilman was allowed to return home, with the instructions to "live as domestic a life as possible…and never touch pen, brush or pencil as long as you live…. She says in her diary that 'I went home, followed those directions rigidly for a month and came perilously near to losing my mind.'"[8]

The claim that the treatment of mental illness ("loss of mind") may make the patient mentally ill ("lose her mind") is a recurrent theme in the history of psychiatry and forms an integral part of the modern concept of mental illness. Today, the theme appears in a pharmacological incarnation: "Miracle drugs" that allegedly cure mental illness and prevent suicide are claimed to cause depression, mania, and suicide.

In 1935, suffering from terminal cancer, Gilman committed suicide by inhaling chloroform. Not until the 1970s, after criticism of the concept of mental illness had gained a foothold in the professional literature and popular media, did *The Yellow Wallpaper* enter the feminist canon. Still, modern feminists interpret Gilman's essay not as an indictment of psychiatric stupidity and brutality but as an expose of "what it was like to live in an emotionally and psychologically restraining society."[9]

2

Personal identities are of two kinds, ascribed and assumed. The identity of mental patient was both imposed on Virginia and appropriated by her. Having been diagnosed as mentally ill when still a child, every time Virginia misbehaved—that is, disturbed, offended, upset others—the diagnosis was revived, and each revival was regarded as a confirmation of its validity. Her "psychotic" rages against Leonard and her dramatic suicide were automatically— conveniently and mindlessly—categorized as manifestations of mental illness.

The core meaning of the term "mental illness," let us not forget, always lay, and continues to lie, in its power to annul ordinary (rational) intentionality. The view that Virginia's mad behavior was unintentional and meaningless (irrational) is shared by all of the compilers and editors of the vast corpus of her work. This "official" attitude toward Virginia's "illness"—firmly held by the best-informed and most sophisticated minds of our age—illustrates the modern faith in the religion of psychiatry.

Leonard never had any doubts that Virginia was insane. Indeed, he married her "knowing" full well that she was mad:

> During the time that I lived in the same house as Virginia in Brunswick Square, and particularly in the months before we married, I became for the first time aware of the menace of nervous or mental breakdown under which she always lived. *I had no experience at all of nervous or mental illness and it was some time before I realized the nature and meaning of it in Virginia. It played a large part in her life and our lives and it was the cause of her death.* If in the following pages I am to give an accurate and understandable account of our life from 1912 to 1941, when she committed suicide, it is necessary at this point that I should explain the nature of her illness. The doctors called it neurasthenia and she had suffered from it all her life.... Superficially the nature of the disease was clear and simple. If Virginia lived a quiet, vegetative life, eating well, going to bed early, and not tiring herself mentally or physically, she remained perfectly well. But if she tired herself in any way, if she was subjected to any severe physical, mental, or emotional strain, symptoms at once appeared which in the ordinary person are negligible and transient, but with her were serious danger signals....

For nearly 30 years I had to study Virginia's mind with the greatest intensity, for it was only by recognizing the first, most tenuous mental symptoms
of fatigue that we could take in time the steps to prevent a serious breakdown. I am sure that, when she had a breakdown, there was a moment when
she passed from what can be rightly called sanity to insanity.[10]

Although Leonard stated that he knew nothing about psychiatry,
he had no trouble understanding the nature of her alleged illness. It
lay, he explained, "in her premises.... She believed, for instance,
that she was not ill.... These beliefs were insane because they were
in fact contradicted by reality."[11] Leonard's view of his wife's
mental state was even darker than that of her psychiatrists and
friends, who viewed her as sometimes sane, sometimes not.
Leonard believed that Virginia was always and permanently insane: "When Virginia was quite well, she would discuss her illness;
she would recognize that she had been mad.... When she was like
that, she was obviously well and sane. *But even then she was not
well and sane in the way in which the vast majority of human beings
are well and sane.*"[12]

Leonard based his opinion that Virginia was always insane on her
attitude toward food, which was the opposite of his and which was a
source of continuous irritation to him, much as Leonard's "animal
appetites" were a constant source of irritation to her. He writes:

[O]ne of the most troublesome symptoms of her breakdowns was a refusal to
eat. In the worst period of the depressive stage, for weeks almost at every
meal one had to sit, often for an hour or more, trying to induce her to eat a few
mouthfuls.... Deep down, this refusal to eat was connected with some strange
feeling of guilt: she would maintain that she was not ill.... This was her
attitude to food when she was in the depths of the depressive stage of her
insanity. *But something of this attitude remained with her always, even
when she appeared to have completely recovered. It was always extremely
difficult to induce her to eat enough food to keep her well.*[13]

Leonard viewed his wife as a woman who would starve to death
unless he fed her or patiently prodded her to feed herself. Time and
again, Leonard returned to the theme of Virginia's culinary frigidity:
"[T]here was always something strange, something slightly irrational in her attitude towards food. It was extraordinarily difficult ever
to get her to eat enough to keep her strong and well."[14]

There was nothing irrational in Virginia's attitude toward food. It
is easy enough to understand it, even if one does not share it. She
was not interested in food and cooking, perhaps was even repelled

by eating, much the same way that she was not interested in sex, or indeed in much of the external world. Leonard had a "healthy, Jewish" interest in food, was proud of it, and was irked by Virginia's lack of interest in eating. He wrote: "It is a strange fact—I have no doubt, discreditable to me, some unsavory juggling between my scruffy ego and sluttish id—that one of the chief things which I remember as connected with the return from those terrible four years of war to peace is chocolate creams."[15]

Convinced that Virginia was psychotically anorexic, Leonard had a maniacal zeal to feed her. No sooner did they marry than he assumed the role of stuffing Virginia. When she had a breakdown in 1913, his campaign to fatten her went into high gear. Leonard weighed Virginia every day and entered the result in his "log." Thus, we learn that in the two-year period between 1913 and 1915, her weight increased from 8 stone/7 pounds to 12 stone/7 pounds, a gain of nearly 50 percent.[16] Virginia's normal weight was said to have been 9 stone. Hence, 8 stone/7 pounds was hardly an alarmingly low figure. One stone is 14 pounds. In pounds, then, Virginia's normal weight was 126 pounds, her lowest weight during this period was 119 pounds, and her highest weight 175 pounds. Thus, Leonard and *his* psychiatrists acted out their therapeutic fantasy of turning Virginia into a stuffed and stupid goose. In their marital relationship, Leonard and Virginia have, in effect, replaced the vaginal-sexual penetration of coitus with the oral-alimentary penetration of feeding.

3

Virginia and Leonard were united in matrimony by mutual repulsion. Each regarded the other as alien and unattractive and couched repulsion in her or his own favorite imagery of the "inhuman." Virginia saw Leonard as "the Jew," alien and disgusting, but vital. Leonard saw Virginia as "the mad genius"—emaciated and insane, but inspired. The theme of the mad-genius Virginia has been widely explored in the extensive Woolf literature and I contribute my share to it in this study. In contrast, the theme of the Jew-aversive Virginia has been systematically downplayed by admirers and critics alike. I want to rectify that neglect.

In 1905, Virginia Stephen wrote to Violet Dickinson: "There are a great many Portuguese Jews on board, and other repulsive objects, but we keep clear of them."[17] In a 1909 notebook, discovered only in 2003, there is a sketch of a Mrs. Loeb: "She is a fat Jewess, aged 56 (she tells her age to ingratiate herself), coarsely skinned, with drooping eyes, and tumbled hair. She fawned upon us, flattered us and wheedled us, in a voice that rubbed away the edges of all her words and had a falling cadence...at dinner she pressed everyone to eat, and feared, when she saw an empty plate, that the guest was criticizing her. Her food, of course, swam in oil and was nasty...[18]

In 1912, Virginia wrote to Madge Vaughan: "Meanwhile, how am I to begin about Leonard? First he is a Jew; second he is 31; third, he spent 7 years in Ceylon, governing natives.... He has no money of his own."[19] In 1923, Virginia, now a Woolf, wrote to Jacques Raverat: "My husband...poor devil, *I make him pay for his unfortunate mistake in being born a Jew.*"[20] In 1930, to Ethel Smyth: "How I hated marrying a Jew—how I hated their nasal voices, and their oriental jewelry, and their noses and their wattles... They can't die...their flesh dries on their bones but still they pullulate, copulate, and amass millions of money."[21]

A month later, again to Ethel Smyth, she wrote: "[H]ere they are [Leonard's relatives], dressed, like all Jews, as if for high tea in a hotel lounge, never mixing with the country, talking nasally, talking incessantly, but requiring at intervals the assurance that I think it really jolly to have them."[22] And in 1932, again to Ethel Smyth: "When the 10 Jews sat around me, silently at my mother-in-laws [sic], tears gathered behind my eyes...imagine eating birthday cake with silent Jews at 11 p.m."[23]

I cite these remarks not to indict Virginia Woolf of anti-Semitism, which would be missing the point. I cite them to indict the Virginia Woolf industry for ignoring the evidence of how deeply revolted Virginia was by Leonard's persona, and for their perpetuating of the fable—fabricated by this ill-fated pair—that they had a perfect marriage, marred only by her madness. Virginia herself strikes this false note with special force in her two suicide notes to Leonard. In the first, probably written on March 18, 1941, she tells him, "I don't think two people could have been happier till this terrible disease came.... I don't think two people could have been happier than we have been."[24] In the second suicide note, dated March 28, the day of her death, she adds, "It is this madness.... All I want to say is that until this disease came on we were perfectly happy."[25] Many students of Virginia Woolf's work and her marriage take these avowals at their face value. The image fits their fantasy about the linkage between madness and genius.

Leonard's confidence in his understanding of the nature and proper treatment of Virginia's mental illness coexisted comfortably with his strident avowal (cited earlier), "I do not know what the present state of knowledge with regard to nervous and mental diseases is in the year 1963; in 1913 it was desperately meager."[26] The issue before us is not what Leonard knew or did not know about mental illness and psychiatry. Rather, it is that he knew very well indeed how to *use psychiatry*. He used it to control and dominate his wife, to deny their marital disharmony, and, during the First World War, to avoid military service.

> He [Maurice Craig] gave me the following certificate, with which, to tell the truth, I did not and do not entirely (medically) agree: "Mr. L. S. Woolf has been known to me for some years and has been previously under my care. Mr. L. S. Woolf is in my opinion entirely unfit for Military Service and would inevitably break down under the conditions of active service. Mr. L. S. Woolf has definite nervous disabilities, and in addition an Inherited Nervous Tremor which is quite uncontrollable.[27]

Leonard viewed Virginia's madness as a life-long affliction that could, at any time, "cause" a fresh "breakdown." In contrast, he viewed his own madness as strictly limited, disabling him from military service only. Years later, Leonard was still indignant about Craig's certifying him as incurably mentally unbalanced; the diagnosis, he maintained, was "medically" mistaken. But Leonard never doubted the accuracy of his own diagnosis of Virginia. She was insane, and he spared no effort to authenticate that verdict. He was also convinced that insanity and creativity were connected, as he stated in his autobiography: "Some pages back I referred to the ancient belief that genius is near allied to madness. I am quite sure that Virginia's genius was closely connected with what manifested itself as mental instability and insanity."[28] Virginia is permanently insane, although her insanity manifests itself only sporadically, in great fits of breakdowns; she is also permanently a genius, although her genius manifests itself only sporadically, in great works of fiction.

The posthumous verdict on Virginia's mental state was sealed by her suicide. A long entry in the *Encyclopedia Britannica* (1973 edition) concludes: "In a recurrence of mental illness...she drowned herself...on March 28, 1941." The statement implies that Virginia did not really intend to take her own life; her deed was something less or other than a rational act, the consequence or result of her mental illness.

Since ancient times, people have recognized that what makes our lives distinctively human, different from the lives of animals, is that our conduct is intentional and goal-directed. It is precisely this conception of man as moral agent—a responsible actor on the stage of life, not an animal exhibiting behavior determined by drives or genes—that the idea of insanity is intended to undermine.[29] The astonishing success of this enterprise in moral deconstruction is illustrated by the fact that the compilers and editors of the vast corpus of Virginia Woolf's work—who rank among the best-informed and most sophisticated persons of our age—unanimously agree that Virginia's behavior during her "breakdowns" was meaningless, in short, that there was no method in her madness. I maintain that the method in her madness was perfectly clear.

Nigel Nicolson, the editor of Virginia's letters, writes: "[Virginia and Leonard] faced the ultimate calamity that she might at any moment go raving mad and turn upon him with vitriolic abuse... There is no record that they, Virginia and Leonard, ever had a serious quarrel, *except when she was insane*...Virginia was mad."[30] This is preposterous interpretation. The truth is that Virginia was repulsed by, and chronically angry at, Leonard. From her point of view, she had perfectly good reasons for being angry at him. Moreover, being "vitriolically abusive" was very much a part of her nature, as everyone who knew her acknowledged. Nevertheless, Nicolson insists that when Virginia was angry, she was "mad," her actions not those of a moral agent: "The truth is that...anything might precipitate a crisis. Her manic-depression (I use the term loosely) could strike with terrifying suddenness."[31]

This is error, not truth. Facts and logic alike contradict Nicolson's interpretation. If *any thing* can precipitate a crisis, then it is logical to conclude that *no one thing* does. Perhaps Virginia herself precipitated the crises. If we were to treat Virginia as an active agent, a manager of her own life, rather than a passive object, the victim of a mental illness, then instead of speaking of a "crisis" being "precipitated," we would speak of Virginia's having a temper tantrum or letting lose her pent-up anger. Virginia's following remark, in a letter she wrote to Janet Case in 1912, shortly after her wedding, supports this interpretation: "...I am quite clear that I shall never really be ill again because with Leonard I get no chance!"[32] The phrase "I get no chance" suggests that she was aware that her "illness" was autogenic, that is, its source lay, ultimately, in herself.[33]

4

Did Virginia view herself as mentally ill or insane? For the most part, yes. Occasionally, she protested feebly. But even then her focus was on ridiculing the incompetence and stupidity of her doctors rather than on claiming moral agency for her conduct. In this way, Virginia displayed the same sort of hypocritical ambivalence about her mental illness that she displayed about her interest in motherhood. She claimed that she wanted to have children, but acquiesced in remaining barren. Sometimes she claimed that she was not mentally ill, but, more often, spoke and wrote about "being ill" and "going insane," and she submitted repeatedly to psychiatric treatments the validity of which she disparaged and rejected.

The endless discussion about Virginia's madness, during her life and since then, would not be possible without the persistent mystification of insanity as an illness and of psychiatry as a medical specialty. Looking at the proceedings from the viewpoint that mental illness is an oxymoron, as I do, I see much of it as serving the function of deceiving others and oneself. All observers of Bloomsbury agree that the only value they truly respected was reason. Like the Jacobins, they were " secular rationalists," just as unreasonable as the "religious irrationalists" they opposed. In his excellent study, *Virginia Woolf and the Real World*, Alex Zwerdling writes: "If Bloomsbury worshiped a god, it was the human brain. This rationalist faith is evident in the title of Goldsworthy Lowes Dickinson's major pacifist work, *War: Its Nature, Cause, and Cure* (1923), with its echo of medical treatises."[34]

Not only were the Bloomsburians fanatical rationalists, they were also devout socialists, their individualist lifestyle notwithstanding. This explains their gullibility about medicine, their naive embrace of medical "treatment" as a political panacea. As late as 1930, Virginia offered this view of the nature of her mental illness: "I believe these illnesses are in my case...partly mystical. Something happens in my mind. It refuses to go on registering impressions. It shuts itself up."[35]

This is gibberish. It was not Virginia's mind, as though it were some sort of electrical instrument, that shut itself off. It was Virginia the person, the moral agent, that shut herself off. Why? Because she could not handle conflict and the intense emotions it generates; because she was a profoundly undisciplined person, a trait for which she paid dearly, and she knew it.

After centuries of mystification, the mystery of madness now runs deep through the grand canyon of Western culture. Even so sophisticated a writer as Zwerdling can't see through Virginia's madness and call a spade a spade: "Woolf's madness was an intensified form of her imaginative life..."[36] Well, of course. But in that case, it was not "madness," not an illness, not a medical problem, and Zwerdling is guilty of being ensnared and ensnaring us in a gross misuse of language. Imagination, by definition, is internal, private, a self-conversation, not directly affecting others. Whereas madness, by definition, is an act, something external, directly affecting others. If Virginia's madness was, as Zwerdling suggests, "an intensified form of her imaginative life"—sometimes, in part, it was that—then it should be called by its proper name: (mis)behavior—fear, frustration, sorrow, helplessness, rage, revenge, and so forth.

Bell's inconsistent and often confused account of Virginia's thoughts concerning her madness mirrors Virginia's inconsistency and ambivalence about the subject. He writes: "It was one of the horrors of Virginia's madness that she was sane enough to recognize her own insanity." In the next paragraph, he contradicts himself: Virginia was "persuaded that...her anxieties and insomnia were due simply to her own faults."[37] The basic task of psychiatry is to deny the validity of this truism and to obfuscate human tragedy by medicalizing it. In this task, psychiatry has been all too successful. Italian critic Francesco Alberoni's summary of the result cannot be improved: "People today talk about health and food. They don't read essays any more that state problems they have to think about.... *We no longer want to understand the process that produces our behavior, individual or social; we want formulas.*"[38] Fake neuroscientists happily supply them: Mind is brain, persons are unhappy and behave badly because they have brain diseases treatable with drugs.

Let us keep in mind that individuals identified as mentally ill and persons eager to dispose of them as mental patients—in our case, Virginia and Leonard Woolf—are engaged in the painful process of decision-making about how to lead their lives, not in an epistemological debate about the medical status of mental illness. Leonard and Virginia avoided that task by using the idea of mental illness and the institution of psychiatry to manipulate each other and their social environment.

Some writers blame Leonard for driving Virginia mad. Notwithstanding the evidence, Roger Poole insists: "She fought to the very last not to be called 'insane,' 'mad,' 'mentally ill.' But always there was Leonard, writing descriptions of her in his secret diary in Tamil... She would not admit that she was insane. And this, of course, quite rightly because she was not."[39]

On February 7, 1912, Virginia writes to Ka Cox, "I've been ill, but I'm practically all right again now. It was a touch of my usual disease, *in the head you know.*"[40] To Vita Sackville-West, on February 7, 1929: "I should have shot myself long ago in one of these illnesses if it hadn't been for him."[41] To Ethel Smyth, on May 1, 1931: "We spent I daresay a hundred pounds when it meant selling my few rings and necklaces to pay them, without any more result than that if I get a pain, go to bed, and eat meat, it goes. No other cure has ever been found—and the disease—well, *all the nerves meet in the spine:* its simple enough."[42] Virginia took to the role of madwoman like the proverbial duck takes to water. In fact, this role was the keystone in the Roman arch of her thoroughly inauthentic, self-deceitful character. She deceived herself not only about her "illness," but also about her longed-for but unfulfilled motherhood and her social-economic status.

In April 1913, three months after her disastrous visit to Sir Henry Head, Virginia lies to herself, and Violet Dickinson to whom she writes: "We aren't going to have a baby but we want to have one, and 6 months in the country or so is said to be necessary first."[43]

Virginia paid dearly for her gutlessness: as a person, she deprived herself of motherhood; as a writer, of moral seriousness. In 1926, she blames herself for not having or exercising more self-control: "A little more self-control on my part, & we might have had a boy of 12, a girl of 10; this always makes me wretched in the early hours."[44] A year later, she writes in her *Diary:* "I'm always angry at myself for not having forced Leonard to take the risk in spite of doctors."[45]

Virginia's self-deceptions about her socioeconomic status followed a similar pattern. Virginia had an inheritance sufficient to live comfortably on the income it generated. This is what allowed her to pursue the life of a writer. Was she grateful for it? No: "I'm one of those who are hampered by the psychological hindrance of owning capital," she wrote in her *Diary.*[46]

Zwerdling observes that "Woolf wanted to think of herself as not privileged but as deprived," and attributes her hypocrisy to "middle-class guilt."[47] However, only economically was Virginia Woolf middle class. Socially, she was very much upper class. Her attitudes toward money and the poor were examples of the liberal-socialist ("Cadillac-Communist") hypocrisy typical of the modern (self-appointed) cultural elite, not expressions of middle-class guilt.

Virginia's problem, as Zwerdling sees it, "was that she could not justify the system that was liberating her. Her solution was to widen the distance between herself and 'the lower orders,' both the servants that released her from household drudgery and the working class that indirectly provided a return on her capital."[48] This is a very benign interpretation of Virginia and Leonard's disdainful and nasty behaviors toward hired help. They related to domestic servants more like Soviet apparatchiks related to members of the expendable lower orders, rather than like rich people in England related to domestic help. Taking Bloomsbury's corrupt political ethos to heart, Julian Bell, Vanessa's son, died fighting for the communists in Spain. Zwerdling quotes Virginia's *Diary* entry: "It is an absurdity how much time L[eonard] and I have wasted talking about servants."[49] It was not an absurdity. It was one of the ways in which they defined their superiority over people who had to earn a living. They were better; they were fighting for International Socialism, World Order, Perpetual Peace.[50]

The *dramatis personae* in Virginia's life were the *crème de la crème* of English literary life—prominent writers, critics, book reviewers. Astoundingly, these eminent literati were satisfied with moronic phrases such as "in the head you know" and "all the nerves meet in the spine" as explanations for Virginia's bad behaviors and bad moods.

Virginia Woolf spent her life on two projects: 1) thinking, talking, and writing about herself, and 2) hiding her true self from others and, more often than not, herself as well. She was most keenly analytical and self-revealing in her novels, as many students of Virginia have noted. As wife and mental patient, she could choose how much, if any, of her intentionality to acknowledge. As writer, she had no such choice: She had to endow her characters with a full measure of the quality that makes a person a human being, namely, intentionality. Hence her superb portraiture of both madman and mad-doctor in *Mrs. Dalloway*, the one novel in which the subject of madness-and-psychiatry occupies center stage.

3

"He shut people up"

1

Of all of Virginia Woolf's novels, I single out for discussion *Mrs. Dalloway*, published in 1925. I do so because it contains an exceptionally perceptive portrait of a typical English psychiatrist of the time, as well as a devastating criticism of psychiatric practice, as valid today as it was then.

Like all of Virginia Woolf's books, *Mrs. Dalloway* is autobiographical, the characters wearing little more than fig leaves to cover their true identity. Septimus Warren Smith, the second principal character in *Mrs. Dalloway*, and Clarissa Dalloway never meet. They occupy parallel universes. As Virginia stated: "I adumbrate here a study of insanity and suicide; the world seen by the sane and the insane side by side."[1] Both Septimus and Clarissa are "sensitive souls" who must protect their inner core from an intrusive-destructive world. Septimus's defenses fail: He is declared insane, and he kills himself. Clarissa's defenses hold: She is sane, a person alienated from herself and others.

Septimus Smith, the husband of Rezia, an Italian woman, is a man for whom "love between man and woman was repulsive.... The business of copulation was filth to him.... But, Rezia said, she must have children. They have been married five years."[2] Virginia's observations of herself and of Leonard, put into the mouths of this couple, are ruthless: "For the truth is (let her ignore it) that human beings have neither kindness, nor faith, nor charity beyond what serves to increase the pleasure of the moment."[3] This is a brutally accurate remark concerning both Virginia's and Leonard's resolute self-centeredness.

Virginia had not forgotten about having babies nor forgiven Leonard for denying them to her: "At tea, Rezia told him that Mrs.

Filmer's daughter was expecting a baby. *She* could not grow old and have no children! She was very lonely, she was very unhappy! She cried for the first time since they were married. Far away, he heard her sobbing...but he felt nothing."[4]

The theme of feeling too much or too little recurs throughout Virginia's life and lunacy. In *Mrs. Dalloway*, Virginia masterfully connects Septimus's "not feeling" ordinary human emotions with his "sins," which he believes are the cause of his misery: "So there was no excuse; nothing whatever the matter, except the sin for which human nature had condemned him to death: that he did not feel."[5]

In *Mrs. Dalloway*, the perspective on mental illness is existential-moral, not medical-scientific. Madness is not "mental illness." It is part and parcel of a moral agent's life and fate, shaped by his decisions and weaknesses ("sins"), and by the decisions and weaknesses of those with whom he colludes in rejecting responsibility for his own life. The fateful step in the career of the mental patient—the moment at which the subject decides to relinquish agency and control over his life and invites others to assume responsibility for him—is evoked with unmatched clarity and precision: "At last, with a melodramatic gesture which he assumed mechanically and with complete consciousness of its insincerity, he dropped his head on his hands. Now he had surrendered; now other people must help him. People must be sent for. He gave in."[6] As she had given in.

Virginia wrote *Mrs. Dalloway* a generation before Sartre characterized the "hysteric" as a liar without a lie, a person victimized by her own "bad faith." Virginia, too, knew very well that the madman is a "liar," that madness is a "lie." Specifically, one of the sins for which Septimus is condemned to death is that he has lied to his wife: "[A]ll the other crimes raised their heads and shook their fingers and jeered and sneered over the rail of the bed in the early hours of the morning...how he had married his wife without loving her; had lied to her... The verdict of human nature on such a wretch was death."[7]

Virginia married Leonard without loving him. She felt guilty, and punished herself by acting mad, being mad, and letting herself be humiliated by Leonard and his carefully chosen psychiatrists. Virginia's portrait of the psychiatrist in *Mrs. Dalloway* can leave no doubt that she understood only too well what psychiatry was, and is, all about. This is her portrait of Sir William Bradshaw, prominent fictional English psychiatrist:

Worshiping proportion, Sir William not only prospered himself but made England prosper, secluded her lunatics, forbade childbirth, penalized despair.... There in the grey room, with the pictures on the wall, and the valuable furniture, under the ground glass skylight, they learnt the extent of their transgressions; huddled up in arm-chairs, they watched him go through, for their benefit, a curious exercise with the arms, which he shot out, brought sharply back to his hip, to prove, if the patient was obstinate, that Sir William was master of his own actions, which the patient was not.[8]

Volumes have been written on psychiatry as a repressive social institution. I have myself contributed to that literature. Virginia Woolf says it all in a few lines: "Naked, defenseless, the exhausted, the friendless received the impress of Sir William's will. He swooped; he devoured. He shut people up. It was this combination of decision and humanity that endeared Sir William so greatly to the relations of his victim."[9] The last two sentences express virtually all of the "problems" of psychiatry, its hidden agendas that set it apart from ordinary medical practice and confuse patients, politicians, and the public. The pithy phrase "He shut people up" expresses the psychiatrist's two core functions: incarcerating the mental patient to protect the family and the public from him; and silencing the mental patient, depriving him of his voice, to maintain the illusion that psychiatric coercion is a medical, not a political, act. In the second sentence, Virginia speaks of Sir William's "victims"; she does not use the term "patient." Lastly, she makes it clear that the psychiatrist is an agent of the denominated patient's family, rendering them a service that "endear[s him] Sir William so greatly to the relations of his victim."

The portrait of psychiatry and the psychiatrist that Virginia paints here rivals that painted a generation earlier by Anton Chekhov in *Ward No. 6*, and would not be matched again until Ken Kesey published *One Flew Over the Cuckoo's Nest*, which, however, focuses on the inmates and their psychiatric prison rather than on the personality or social role of the psychiatrist as judge and jailer.

One wonders what Leonard thought when he read *Mrs. Dalloway*. How could he not have concluded that the portrait of psychiatry presented in it revealed Virginia's view of psychiatry? And if that is what he concluded—if that idea so much as occurred to him—why did he not confront Virginia *and himself* with its logical implication, namely: Why go to a doctor if you are not sick? Why go to a physician whom you do not respect? Why seek a type of medical treatment in which you do not believe?

There is no evidence that Leonard ever put these questions either to Virginia or himself. Virginia, Leonard, and everyone around them avoided asking the relevant related questions, for example, What is mental illness? Are psychiatrists curing disease or controlling deviance? Still, *they had to answer these questions, if not verbally, then behaviorally.* And answer them they did. Leonard, the rationalist, was consistent. He knew that mental illness is like any other illness, and that if the patient did not cooperate in its cure, then she had to be coerced. Virginia, the "irrationalist," was inconsistent. As a writer, she knew that there was no such thing as mental illness and that psychiatrists were pseudomedical inquisitors and wardens; but as a non-writer—as wife, sister, citizen—she acted as if she accepted the reality of mental illness and the legitimacy of psychiatry as a medical specialty.

Virginia was right when she maintained that there is no such thing as mental illness, as she implies in *Mrs. Dalloway*; that (mis)behaviors, such as she exhibited, were, in an important sense, the subject's own "faults"; that so-called mental illnesses are existential-moral problems; that, in short, she lacked integrity, not mental health. But she did not *mean* any of this. *Mrs. Dalloway* was just a "story." If ever evidence were needed that insight does not "cure mental illness," here it is. The reason is obvious: One cannot "cure" mental illness—an autogenic "illness"—against the wish of the patient. Virginia did not want to renounce the role of mental patient in 1913; was not prepared to renounce it in 1923; and still held on to it tightly in 1941, when she killed herself.

As a thought experiment, let us ask what Virginia could have done after marrying Leonard and realizing that she made a huge mistake. She could have scrutinized—interrogated herself about—the problems she was trying to solve by acting crazy. This would have required her to confront the sort of matrimonial bond she and Leonard were forging and the seriousness of the sentence of childlessness that her husband was determined to impose on her; to examine the truth inherent in her self-blame, with its source in her self-indulgent preoccupation with herself; and to challenge the wisdom of submitting herself to a type of psychiatric care in the value of which she profoundly, and rightly, disbelieved. Virginia chose not to do any of these things.

All this is idle speculation. If Virginia could have made such choices, she would not have been the person she was. Again and again, Virginia asserted that her madness had "saved" her. The path of self-emancipation via self-responsibility did not lead to the destination she sought to reach. Virginia, her family, Leonard, and their psychiatrists colluded with one another in going down another road, the well-traveled superhighway called "mental illness." This choice had many advantages for all concerned (or else they would not have chosen it). Most importantly, it enabled them, whenever they so chose, to ignore the disturbing meaning of Virginia's behavior by ascribing it to her mental illness. This, in turn, enabled them to regard Virginia as "mad" and "treat" her "illness," instead of taking seriously the tragedy this "explanation" concealed. Virginia could settle down to being a mad genius; Leonard, to being married to a madwoman writer; Vanessa, to having a mad sister.

Virginia knew very well what she was doing when she submitted to psychiatric treatment and avoided psychoanalysis. In 1917, Freud wrote, "Psychiatry...can only say with a shrug: 'Degeneracy, hereditary disposition, constitutional inferiority!' Psychoanalysis sets out to explain these uncanny disorders." Comparing the mentally ill patient to an absolute ruler who does not want to know the truth about the people he tyrannizes, he enjoins the "sufferer" to look inward: "You behave like an absolute ruler who is content with the information supplied him by his highest officials and never goes among the people to hear their voice. Turn your eyes inward, look into your own depths, learn first to know yourself! Then you will understand why you were bound to fall ill; and perhaps you will avoid falling ill in the future."[10] That was not what Virginia wanted. She preferred to collude with psychiatrists in denying the meaning of her "illness."

2

After World War II, Virginia's mind was quickly exhumed and submitted to posthumous psychiatric study and diagnosis. Not surprisingly, each result depended on the point the commentator wished to make. Some wanted to rehabilitate her by claiming that she was not mad. Others wanted to use her life and death as evidence of the reality of mental illness as a fatal disease.

The Unknown Virginia Woolf, by Roger Poole (1939-2003), a distinguished English literary theorist, is a major work devoted to proving that Virginia was sane. Poole begins by noting that Virginia's married name is an "existential oxymoron," a violation of her real self.[11] I agree. As an author, she could have retained her distinguished family name or used it as a middle name. She did neither. Poole's incisive remark shows us that Virginia was not much of a feminist and that those who celebrate her as such do violence to the facts. She was a conformist, an exhibitionist, and, as she herself acknowledged, a first class snob and coward. To be sure, she criticized male domination and psychiatric slavery, but she did so cautiously, elliptically—not directly and forcefully in the tradition of the great English feminists and abolitionists.

Poole's argument derails when he asks, "Was Virginia Woolf 'mad'?" and sets out to show that she was not because her mad behavior had meaning.[12] As Sartre said, "The Jew is one whom other men consider a Jew; that is the simple truth from which we must start."[13] Similarly, a mentally ill person is one whom others consider mentally ill; we deal here with the language of stigma, not the language of nosology.

The ability to find meaning in madness—to attribute sense to the "senseless" behavior of the mentally ill person, whether that ability is exercised by Shakespeare, Freud, or anyone else—forms no part of the criteria that psychiatrists use to diagnose mental illness. Psychiatrists do have criteria for what counts as a mental illness, and it does no good to pretend they do not. Accordingly, it is reasonable to reject the psychiatric perspective on behaviors called mental illnesses as conceptually false and morally objectionable. But it is unreasonable to accept the psychiatric perspective and argue that because there is method in a particular patient's madness, he is not mad. This is precisely the mistake the defenders of Virginia's good psychiatric name make.[14]

Poole complains: "When I read Professor Bell's biography, I was puzzled by the failure to offer any evidence for the alleged 'madness' of his subject."[15] Evidently, Poole was not aware that there is no biological test for mental illness. There is only "expert" psychiatric opinion, which was, and is, unanimous in declaring Virginia to be mad. Poole does not question the nature or reality of mental illness. Instead, he argues that Virginia was not mentally ill: "Virginia's mental condition was not so much 'ill' as anguished... She needed subtle *treatment*, she needed existential, even theological, aid. What she did not need was rest, or food, or sequestration from the world."[16] Poole flirts with the idea that mental illness is a myth, but shies away from it. He falls into the same trap that Leonard and the psychiatrists had fallen into, a trap that Virginia had laid for them, deliberately or unwittingly. He treats Virginia as if she were a sick infant who did not know what she needed, and who, even if she did, could not secure the needed—"existential" or "theological" help—for herself. But she was not a child. She was not helpless. She was an adult, she was intelligent, and she had her own money. She could have rejected the psychiatric "help" her family secured for her and sought help from other quarters, say a Freudian or Jungian therapist. Or she could have eschewed formal "therapy" and tried to help herself in some other way she considered appropriate for what "ailed" her. She did none of these things. Instead, she embraced the role of mental patient and repeatedly submitted to the psychiatric "help" others eagerly secured for her.

Sadly, even so sophisticated an author as Poole is confused, and confuses the reader, about the fundamental distinctions between psychiatry and psychoanalysis, psychiatrist and psychoanalyst. After tracing Virginia's personal problems to what he thinks are its sources and demonstrating the method in her madness, Poole protests: "[I]f a psychiatrist wants to understand what is wrong with his patient, surely the first thing he should be attentive to is the meanings the patient attached to words."[17] This is hopelessly mistaken: *The psychiatrist does not want to understand what ails his patient; he wants to misunderstand it.* The last thing he wants is to understand, in ordinary language, "what is wrong with his patient." Rather, he wants to misunderstand it by translating personal anguish and turmoil into the medical-diagnostic terms that comprise the language of lunacy.

In *All That Summer She Was Mad*, Stephen Trombley, editor of the journal *Books & Issues*, defends Virginia Woolf's sanity in much the same way as Poole does. He simplistically labels Virginia a "female victim of male medicine," asks, "Was Virginia Woolf mad?", and answers: "Many critics, including her biographer, Quentin Bell, and her husband, Leonard, have said that she was. Yet these are lay critics, who have no knowledge of *medical science....* To my knowledge, no one has made a *truly scientific medical study of Virginia Woolf. Until concrete evidence is produced, it is irresponsible to speak of her as having been mad.*"[18]

There is no such thing as "concrete evidence" of madness—there never was, and there never will be. Madness is not that sort of "thing." Trombley writes: "To my knowledge, no one has made a *truly scientific medical study of Virginia Woolf.*" This is the sort of nonsense to which ignorance of medicine together with belief in mental illness inevitably lead. Virginia is dead. She cannot *now* be examined medically. Furthermore, a *"truly scientific medical study of Virginia Woolf"* would entail a thorough autopsy of her corpse, which would be useless, as madness cannot be diagnosed by examining corpses. Also, Trombley knows that the view that Virginia was mentally ill was no mere lay assumption, that the most highly qualified physicians in London repeatedly diagnosed and treated her as mad.

Trombley takes R. D. Laing as his psychiatric guide and guru: "Borrowing from Laing, my programme of phenomenological analysis may be defined briefly: the reconstruction of the other person's experience from his own point of view."[19] Like Laing, Trombley ignores the epistemological status and legal significance of the concept of madness. Instead, he sets out to show that Virginia's *behavior was not senseless; hence she was not insane.*

This is a non sequitur. Virginia is considered insane because she behaved in ways regarded as the classical manifestations of mental illness. She "heard voices." She *said* she was "mad" or "going mad." She tried to kill herself. She died by suicide. In short, she fulfilled the criteria that modern psychiatry and society use to diagnose a person as mentally ill. Trombley acknowledges but dismisses all this: "All of these symptoms can be explained and all of them have meaning.... It is true that Virginia behaved violently toward her family and her nurses because she felt she was being persecuted."[20] This is excusing Virginia's behavior, not demonstrating her sanity—*a priori*, an impossible task. Trombley's effort to explain away Virginia's attitude toward food nicely illustrates just how impossible it is.

Trombley acknowledges Virginia's food-avoidance, calls it "the problem of food," and notes that this behavior is regarded as a typical symptom of anorexia nervosa. He writes: "But to accept this diagnosis would be to confuse the issue. In Virginia's case, the significance of the problem is existential, sexual, ontological."[21] This is true not just in Virginia's case, and not just about anorexia, but about virtually every kind of so-called mentally abnormal behavior. Obviously, self-starvation may be categorized as religious ritual (fasting), mental illness (anorexia nervosa), or political protest (hunger strike), depending on how the subject presents it and how we choose to view and respond to it.

Instead, Virginia's entourage split her into two persons, one sane, the other insane. Worse, they denied that they did the splitting, attributing it instead to the disease they called "madness." After thus dividing Virginia, they never doubted that her sane self was responsible for her brilliant works and her love of Leonard, and that her insane self was not responsible for her brutal words and hatred of Leonard. But how did they know when she was sane and when she was insane? When she wrote novels, she was sane; when she starved herself and was angry at Leonard, she was insane.

Categorizing and calling Virginia's aggressive, meddling condemnation of pleasure in eating "the problem of food" represents a radical depersonalization of voluntary behavior and a refusal to recognize Virginia as a responsible agent. There was no "problem of food." The "problem" was Virginia's socially deviant attitude toward eating: "Virginia was always critical of her friends' behavior at table. Her sensitivity on this point was perhaps connected with her own phobias about eating, phobias which, when she was ill, could make her starve herself and, at ordinary times, make her always very reluctant to take second helping of anything. George Duckworth, Julian Bell, Kingsley Martin were all, at various times, severely condemned for eating with too little grace and too much enthusiasm."[22]

Trombley's comment about this account is: "Towards the end of his biography he [Bell] takes up the food problem [sic] for the last time, and so dismisses it."[23] It is Trombley, not Bell, who dismisses evidence and analysis. Virginia had a right to condemn and reject pleasure in eating and in heterosexual coitus, but she had no right to expect others to feel and behave as she did. That behavior does not make her mad; it only makes her boorish, meddling, and nasty.

Virginia never made a serious effort to reject psychiatric interference in her life, never insisted on living her life without psychiatry. Ironically, she believed in *mental illness* more strongly, and certainly more naively, than did her psychiatrists. Both Sir George Henry Savage (1842-1921) and Sir Henry Head (1861-1940) *recognized that insane behavior is not meaningless and that insanity is not a bona fide medical illness.* In 1905, Savage wrote: "I would repeat here...*the statement that there is no such thing as insanity.* Insanity, mental disorder, depends as much on the surroundings as on the individual's bodily condition."[24]

Head distinguished between medical (bodily) disease and non-disease, which he called "functional disorder": In Trombley's words, "The former involves organic change...while the latter involves a disturbance of the patient's conceptualization of the world."[25] In 1920, Head wrote: "Face to face with the patient, it is futile to waste time in considering whether he is a case of neurasthenia, psychasthenia, anxiety neurosis, or hysteria. The war has unfortunately increased the universal love of labels.... Diagnosis of the psycho-neuroses is an individual investigation: *they are not diseases, but morbid activities of the personality which demand to be understood.*"[26] Head spoke of "activities of the personality which demand to be understood." Now, correct psychiatric practice demands that the psychiatrist drug those "activities of the personality" out of existence, lest he be charged with medical negligence for failure to treat his patient's "brain disease."

Unquestionably, Virginia was victimized by her doctors, just as she was victimized by her husband. But that is only one part of the story. The other part, which Trombley misses, involves the whys and ways in which Virginia and Leonard used psychiatry and psychiatrists to orchestrate their own lives, as madwoman-wife-writer and nurse-husband-manager.

Trombley's psychiatric rehabilitation of Virginia Woolf vitiates its own important truth. One of Trombley's aims is to criticize psychiatry, particularly its historical enmity toward women. But that cannot be done by selective interpretation. The fact is that Virginia collaborated and colluded with psychiatrists in creating her dual identity as madwoman and artist, in much the same way that, say, Joan of Arc collaborated and colluded with the Church-State of her day in creating her dual identity as witch and patriot. The conversion of a martyred apostate into a saint does not hold the Church up to the obloquy it deserves in this matter, nor does the posthumous conversion of a person diagnosed as mad into one certified as sane hold psychiatry up to the obloquy it deserves.[27] Instead of weakening the authority of religion and psychiatry, these tactics only reinforce their legitimacy. It is more truthful, and I hope in the long run more useful, to argue that there is no witchcraft and no mental illness than to consecrate Joan as a saint and certify Virginia as sane.

3

The madness and marriage of Virginia Woolf have provided a golden opportunity for some feminists to display their misandry, the mirror of misogyny, in all its mindlessness. The most extreme misandrist interpretation of the life and work of Virginia Woolf is Irene Coates's study, *Who's Afraid of Leonard Woolf? A Case for the*

Sanity of Virginia Woolf.[28] Coates, a prominent Australian playwright, devotes much of her book to lambasting authors who claim that Virginia was insane. Unfortunately, her thesis is marred by the same mistake that characterizes the works she criticizes: She, too, accepts uncritically the conceptual apparatus and idiom of psychiatry. Her failure to consider what madness is, why some people are called "mentally ill," and why such persons are incarcerated by doctors, vitiates her core thesis that Virginia was sane.

Coates's screed is a piece of ill-conceived feminist fury, untroubled by the requirements of consistency, logic, or truth. She simultaneously asserts that Virginia Woolf was not mad, that she was driven mad by Leonard, and that madness imparted a "superior sanity" to her and made her the genius she was. Coates's animus toward Leonard knows no bounds. She holds him responsible for single-handedly "driving" his wife mad and for her suicide. Her admiration for Virginia is similarly unrestrained. Coates argues not only that Virginia was the embodiment of sanity until Leonard managed to drive her mad, but also that after having been driven insane Virginia was saner than ever: "Soon after their marriage Virginia suffered two major nervous breakdowns. She found a way of escaping into an altered state of consciousness within which she discovered a deeper level of creativity: indeed, an *enriched sanity.*"[29]

As we have seen, a few months after Virginia and Leonard wed, Sir Henry Head declared Virginia mentally unfit to have children. That evening, Virginia made a serious suicidal gesture. Coates's version of this event illustrates her prosecutorial eagerness to exaggerate the case against Leonard: "Returning to the house and putting Virginia to bed that evening, after their visit to the doctors [Savage and Head], Leonard went out.... In doing so, he left the box containing Virginia's Veronal (her usual sleeping pills, a type of barbiturate) unlocked and open by her side. Alone, Virginia took a lethal overdose of *100 grams*, and then lapsed into a coma."[30] After some discussion, Coates adds: "My alternative title for this book is *Getting Away With Murder.* However, no thanks to Leonard, this is not what happened in 1913."[31]

Let me set the record straight. Veronal, also known as Barbital (diethylbarbituric acid) is a barbiturate sedative. "Overdoses induce protracted sleep in proportion to the amount taken. Two or two and one-half drams will produce death, though a fatal ending is slow in occurring. Sleep has been prolonged ten days with recovery."[32] Prior to the war on drugs, barbiturates were the most widely used sleep-inducing agents. The usual dose was 5-10 grains or 0.32-0.64 grams. *Coates asserts that Virginia ingested 100 grams, that is, almost a quarter of a pound of Veronal, an impossibly large quantity to ingest.*

Moreover, it is not true, as Coates states, that on that particular occasion (and many times later) Leonard made no effort to prevent Virginia's killing herself. He had arranged for Ka Cox to stay with Virginia. Cox quickly discovered that Virginia had taken Veronal and was in a deep sleep. Virginia's stomach was washed out, and that was the medical end of the matter. Existentially, it was the real beginning of Virginia's being cast so deeply in the role of insane person that there was no escaping from it—not that she wanted to escape it.

Perversely, Coates uses Virginia's not having died from a drug overdose as one more reason for attacking Leonard. "From now on, Leonard took total responsibility for Virginia. *He refused to have her certified as insane.*"[33] Would Coates think better of Leonard if he had committed Virginia? If he had divorced her? Coates explains: "Leonard never understood that her so-called madness was in fact an extended and enriched sanity...she became an autonomous person."[34] But only a few pages later, Coates quotes Virginia's declaring this: "I was so tremblingly afraid of my own insanity that I wrote *Night and Day* mainly to prove to my own satisfaction that I could keep entirely off that dangerous ground. I wrote it, lying in bed, allowed to write for only one half hour a day."[35]

Coates is right about one thing and about that she is more right than any other writer about Virginia—namely, the insurmountable obstacle that Leonard's Jewishness posed to the marriage. Coates aptly refers to Leonard's novel, *The Wise Virgins*, in which Harry, one of the protagonists, addresses his friend Trevorand: "I admire your pale women with their white skins and fair hair, but I despise them. / Do most Jews feel like that? / All of them—all of them."[36]

In her effort to rehabilitate Virginia Woolf, Coates debases her, much as do the writers she criticizes, especially Quentin Bell. Bell excuses Virginia's misbehavior by attributing it to mental illness. Coates excuses it by blaming it on Leonard. In either case, Virginia is denied agency, deprived of responsibility for her behavior, and diminished as a person.

4

"My madness saved me"

1

How did Virginia Woolf view her so-called breakdowns? Did she regard herself as a person afflicted with a chronic mental illness? Sometimes she did, and sometimes she did not; she wanted the advantages of both sanity and insanity, and the disadvantages of neither.

We know that Virginia held psychiatrists in contempt, yet repeatedly submitted to their care; and that she respected and was friends with psychoanalysts, but carefully avoided seeking their professional help. In 1904, she wrote to Violet Dickinson: "My life is a constant fight against Doctors [sic] follies, it seem to me."[1] Still, she acquiesced to psychiatric attention for the rest of her life, but avoided psychoanalytic assistance. Why? Because she did not fear psychiatry but feared psychoanalysis, and because she wanted to avail herself of the benefits that the role of chronic mental patient offered.

The psychiatrist posed no threat to Virginia's soul. The great psychiatrist Sir William in *Mrs. Dalloway* was a bungler, not interested in the soul and its terrors. It is important to remember this because the modern reader, especially if he is "psychoanalytically sophisticated," thinks of the psychiatric physician, as contrasted with a regular doctor or surgeon, as a person eager to know his patient as a person. This is generally not true today, was not true in Virginia's day, and was not true in the days when psychiatry's most celebrated madman, Judge Daniel Paul Schreber, was treated by Paul Flechsig, one of the most prominent German psychiatrists of that era. In his famous *Memoirs*, Schreber complained: "[Flechsig] *did not understand the living human being* and had no need to understand him, because...he dealt only with corpses."[2]

Unlike Septimus Smith, Virginia knew how to defend herself against men such as Sir William or Sir Henry (Head), indeed how to manipulate them. All she needed to do was eat and pretend she was getting "better," and they would be happy to leave her alone. The last thing an English luminary of lunacy wanted was to *understand* a woman like Virginia Woolf. He was confident that he already *knew* all there was to know about her: She was the daughter of Sir Leslie Stephen and the niece of Sir James Fitzjames Stephen, both eminent Victorians. She was insane. Her insanity was hereditary and incurable. What else was there to know? The psychiatrist could not cure her. But he knew how to do his job, which was to treat her medically—ordering her to rest and eat and telling her how to live her life. And he knew how to treat her socially—impersonally, with the distance and respect due to a highborn English woman. It was psychoanalysis that Virginia feared and avoided, even though her brother, sister-in-law, and some of her closest friends were psychoanalysts.

2

We all seek intimacy and, fearing the loss of our independence, also avoid it. A close human relationship may be a source of security or a threat or both.

The kinds of relationships in which we engage are, in part, structured by the society in which we live. In the modern West, two of the relationships in which intimacy was, until recently, expected to develop were matrimony and medicine (especially psychotherapy). Virginia's choices for both of these relationships strongly support the view that she was afraid of being "known" and thus violated: She chose for both her husband and her therapist insensitive individuals, incapable of understanding others, especially if they were "different" or "irrational." In my view, Virginia used marriage and madness as masks behind which she hid, the better to be able to pursue her ambitions to write, be famous, and be left alone.

A mask worn over a long period of time tends, however, to become a part of the wearer's face. Virginia's *acting married* and *acting mad* became her *marriage* and her *madness*, each both protecting and endangering her. Especially when mad, she rejected Leonard and being cast into the role of mental patient. Yet, she often spoke of being protected by Leonard and, in her suicide note to him, she wrote: "What I want to say is I owe all the happiness of my life to you."[3] In a letter to Jacques Raverat in 1924 she declared: "My madness saved me."[4] From what did madness save Virginia? From putting her money where her mouth was: from reconciling her knowledge of herself with her personal conduct.

In 1933 Virginia wrote in her diary: "I've been reading Faber on Newman; compared his account of a nervous breakdown; the refusal of some part of the mechanism; is that what happens to me?... No. I think the effort to live in two spheres—the novel, and life—is a strain.... I only want walking and perfectly spontaneous childish life with Leonard and the accustomed life when I'm writing at full tilt."[5]

Alfred Adler called this sort of denial of what one knows to be true while pretending it is not, the "life-lie," and regarded such self-deception as the basic "cause" of mental illness.[6] Virginia's determination to divide her existence into two separate spheres—literature and life, neither on speaking terms with the other—is a dramatic example of such a "life-lie." Herein lies the key to resolving the seeming paradox between her rejection of psychiatric treatment in her fiction, and her acceptance of it in her life.

In *A Room of One's Own*, Virginia remarks, perhaps a bit wistfully, "I find myself saying briefly and prosaically that it is much more important to be oneself than anything else."[7] But it is impossible to be oneself if one is profoundly dissatisfied with one's self. In principle, Virginia could have chosen to obey the Socratic-Shakespearean injunction "To thyself be true." However, obeying that injunction requires both a willingness to search one's soul and a firm resolve to fashion a coherent self to which one can be joyfully true. Virginia rejected this course of action, which perhaps also accounts for why she never chose to seek help from a wise friend or humane psychotherapist who might have helped her to reconcile the warring factions within herself. Instead, especially after her marriage to Leonard, she chose to alternate between two roles: sane writer and mad wife. When writing, she focused on the intentionality of human beings, including persons said to be mad or those caring for them. The result was that in her fiction, Virginia expressed precisely the sort of insight into mental illness and psychiatry to which she blinded herself—but not completely—in her personal life. On June 22, 1930, she wrote to Ethel Smyth: "My terror of life has always kept me in a nunnery. And then I married, and then my brains went up in a shower of fireworks. As an experience, madness is terrific I can assure you, and not to be sniffed at; and in its lava I can still find most of the things I write about."[8]

Virginia is ambiguous about whether madness befalls her or is begot by her. It is a bit of both. Recognition of this duality—of activity and passivity, intentionality and non-intentionality—must be part of an accurate account of what "madness" is.[9] Freud's phrase, "the return of the repressed" obscures the intentionality of the mad person. It makes it seem as if "the repressed" returns unexpectedly, like a long lost relative, without any participation by the subject: The "patient" is a passive "victim" of his repression, which returns as a "symptom," for example, "hearing voices," one of Virginia's symptoms. This is not true. The individual as a moral agent always chooses his *style* of behavior, whether in sanity, insanity, art, or work. Once a person adopts a style, not every *specific feature* of his behavior needs to be deliberately selected; some are culturally prefabricated (for example, hearing the voice of Jesus or Mohammed). Virginia was determined not to be violated by being "known." She did not want anyone to be intimate with her or to know her intimately. That is why she chose to express her real sentiments and thoughts as fiction or as mental symptom, neither of which was real for her husband, family, friends, or her psychiatrists. For these paragons of reality-testing, when Virginia manifestly raged against her husband, she was not *attacking Leonard*; she suffered from an *attack of madness*. When she painted a portrait of a fictional psychiatrist as a pompous, ignorant, and meddling fool, she was *not criticizing psychiatry*; she was *producing a work of art*.

It is not surprising that psychiatrists as well as lay persons are fond of connecting madness and art, the most effective way we human beings have *for taming painful communications by de-meaning* them—categorizing them as either madness or art. Ironically, the more severe the "symptom," the more obvious its meaning, and the more stubbornly psychiatrists, and people generally, insist that it is meaningless. This is especially true for murder in the family. For example, when a mother kills her children, her husband, parents, psychiatrists, prosecutor, defense lawyer, judge, jury, and the press reassure one another and themselves that the deed was a manifestation of mental illness.

3

The subject of Virginia Woolf's avoidance of psychoanalytic help has received surprisingly little attention in the vast literature on her psychiatric problems. Virginia was well aware of the fundamental differences between psychiatry and psychoanalysis. To be sure, the distinction between them was much clearer in England in the 1920s than it is the United States today, as the correspondence between Alix and James Strachey dramatically illustrates. Both Stracheys sought personal analysis to qualify and gain status as lay analysts. On January 27, 1925, Alix—being psychoanalyzed in Berlin by Karl Abraham—wrote to her husband:

> I don't quite share your glowing views as to the prospects [for lay analysts], a.) if "lay" analysts are encouraged to analyze children (which means human beings up to 16) what earthly ground will medical analysts have for deprecating adult analyses of them? b.) From your account I think that the medicos will find they are shorthanded at their clinic. c.) There are Dr. Sachs & a Dr. Mueller, neither medical, in full swing here. It's true they're not in evidence at the Clinic, but they get patients. But America is bad, I admit.[10]

But the Stracheys themselves were caught in the deceptions of the psychoanalytic vocabulary, which they made no attempt to transcend. On February 9, 1925, Alix wrote: "I had a non-analytical conversation with Dr. Abraham today about the length of my analysis. He wanted to know how long I should be able to go on with it. I said indefinitely, i.e., till I was well."[11] What did Alix think ailed her? Not her homosexuality, with which she was well satisfied, although analysts had a rather dismal view of it. Nor her anorexia—she was much thinner than Virginia—which she also had no intention of abandoning. Alix does not say what she wants to be cured of or how she will know that she is "well." A few days later, in characteristically Bloomsbury style, she wrote: "I *do* think the English splendid in their madness."[12]

Although Virginia cultivated the myth that she was ignorant about psychoanalysis, she knew a good deal about it. When she wrote about psychoanalysis, she obviously did not mean psychiatry; and when she portrayed a psychiatrist, as she does in *Mrs. Dalloway*, it is clear that she was not painting the picture of a psychoanalyst. For anyone who pays attention to what psychiatrists and psychoanalysts *do*, the distinction between psychiatry and psychoanalysis is, and has always been, obvious.[13]

"Know thyself" (Oracle of Delphi). "The unexamined life is not worth living" (Socrates). "To thine ownself be true" (Shakespeare, *Hamlet*, Act I, Scene 3). "Though this be madness, yet there is method in't" (Shakespeare, *Hamlet*, Act II, Scene 2). These existential-moral precepts form the foundation of psychoanalysis. Whatever may be said in criticism of psychoanalysis, and however much its founding principles have been corrupted by modern American medicalized "psychoanalysis," this much must be conceded on Freud's behalf.

The (ostensible) psychoanalytic goal of understanding human behavior—normal *and* abnormal—was responsible for the initial humanistic thrust of Freud's enterprise and for the following it brought him. Unfortunately, his vision and his formulation were fatally flawed. The flaw lay in what he really meant when he spoke of "explain[ing] these uncanny disorders." He meant "explaining" them in terms that would enrich and satisfy him and make him famous, not in terms that would enrich and satisfy the patient by enabling him to assume control of the meaning-making of his life.

Virginia Woolf inverted the injunction of the Oracle of Delphi. She pursued self-knowledge *the better to deceive herself.* Joanne Greenberg—Frieda Fromm-Reichmann's famous patient and the author of *I Never Promised You a Rose Garden*"[14]—was familiar with this life tactic ("defense mechanism"). She wrote: "Self-deceit is a strong fort; / It will last a lifetime. / Self-truth is a lightning bolt lost as I grasp it. / And the fires that it strikes can raze my house."[15] This is true only for a life built on lies, a house of cards soaked in the gasoline of deception and self-deception. Virginia knew that engaging in psychoanalysis would require entering into a truthful conversation with herself, and this she had no intention of doing. In my opinion, that is why she avoided seeking psychoanalytic help.

We know that Virginia was obsessed with protecting herself—her body, her person, her soul. For her, being "known"—by a psychoanalyst or anyone else, perhaps even herself—meant being penetrated and violated. She was afraid of, and repelled by, Freud's passion to "unmask" his subject, to "know" him. That was not what Virginia wanted. She preferred to collude with psychiatrists in denying the meaning of her "illness."

It is important to remember that, in Europe, unlike in America, psychoanalysis was not a part of psychiatry. Many leading psychoanalysts—Anna Freud, Melanie Klein, Erik Erikson, Bruno Bettelheim—were not physicians. However, since the 1960s, especially in the United States, the cultural-economic status of psychoanalysis has undergone a profound transformation. Today, the authorities who speak for psychoanalysis insist that it is an integral part of psychiatry, a form of medical treatment that ought to be covered by insurance on a par with treatment for broken bones.

Both Virginia and Leonard Woolf knew many psychoanalysts and were exceptionally knowledgeable about psychoanalysis. They founded, owned, and operated the Hogarth Press and were the first publishers of Freud's works in English. Virginia's brother Adrian and his wife Karin were both psychoanalysts. James Strachey, the authorized translator of Freud's works, and his wife Alix were analysts, members of the Bloomsbury group, and close friends of the Woolfs. In 1914, Leonard read Freud's *Interpretation of Dreams* and reviewed *The Psychopathology of Everyday Life*.

Quentin Bell recognizes the importance that the choice of mental healers played in Virginia's life. He speculates that "if he [Leonard] had read Freud two years earlier [that is, in 1912], Virginia's medical history might have been different." He then dismisses the thought with the remark that "analysts are usually reluctant to treat patients who have actually been mad."[16] This is not true. Many analysts, then and since, treated persons considered "mad" (by their relatives or psychiatrists). The condition Bell calls "being actually mad" is, of course, not a phenomenon. It is a vague term used in literary, medical, psychiatric, and legal contexts. Bell ought to have scrutinized its meaning and function. Typically, people attach the term to individuals whom they regard as embarrassing, strange, or "dangerous to themselves or others." Sometimes, they attach it to others whom they simply regard as eccentric; and sometimes, casually, to themselves, as when a person exclaims, "I must have been mad when..."

Bell accepts psychiatry as a bona fide medical enterprise and views his aunt as a childlike person whose care was the responsibility of her family and doctors. But Virginia was not a child. She was an adult, an author, a famous writer, and a successful publisher. In *Mrs. Dalloway*, she cogently criticizes psychiatry and presents a nonmedical (existential-moral) perspective on mental illness. The question remains: Why did she never consider taking such an approach to her own problems?

4

In his autobiography, Leonard Woolf writes: "In the decade before 1924, in the so-called Bloomsbury circle there was great interest in Freud and psycho-analysis, and the interest was extremely serious."[17] After founding the Hogarth Press in 1917, Virginia read, or at least examined, everything they published, which included Freud's *Collected Papers*. She also had access to information about psychoanalysis through her brother and sister-in-law, and through the Stracheys. On January 21, 1918, Virginia writes in her diary: "Lytton Strachey...gave us an amazing account of the British Sex Society which meets at Hampstead... 50 people of both sexes and various ages discussed without shame such questions as the deformity of Dean Swift's penis...self abuse...incest between parent and child when they are both unconscious of it, was their main theme, derived from Freud. I think of becoming a member."[18]

Content and tone both suggest the curiosity of the would-be acolyte. Her next diary reference to Freud, dated November 21, 1918, shows that she was a quick study. In two sentences, she captures one of the most essential features of psychoanalysis, namely, that *it is not a medical activity*: "James [Strachey], billed at the 17 Club to lecture on 'Onanism,' proposes to earn his living as an exponent of Freud in Harley Street. For one thing, *you can dispense with a degree*."[19]

Although not formally educated, Virginia Woolf was very smart. She instantly recognized the importance of a person's being able to practice psychoanalysis without being a medical doctor, without a medical license. Perhaps she concluded (as many others have since) that if a psychoanalytic practitioner could be a layperson, and "therapy" consisted only of listening and speaking, then *ipso facto* the diseases being treated were fake illnesses. What, then, were psychoanalysts doing? They were ferreting out their patients' secrets, especially sexual secrets, and trying to influence their clients to change their behavior.

In 1919, Adrian and Karin Stephen were preparing to become psychoanalysts. In a letter to Vanessa, dated June 18, 1919, Virginia wrote: "Well, I dropped in on Adrian and Karin the other night... They've given up philosophy, social reform, law, and all the rest of it; they're going into practice together as Psychoanalysts."[20] Virginia could observe the cultishness of the developing psychoanalytic movement from up close and rightly did not like what she saw.

By 1921, Virginia had arrived at a considered position on psychoanalysis. She opposed it as an invasion of the personality likely to make the patient worse. On September 2, 1921, she wrote to Janet Case, "The last people I saw were James and Alix, fresh from

Freud...James puny and languid—such is the effect of 10 months psychoanalysis."[21] On May 12, 1923, she wrote in her diary:

Adrian is altogether broken up by psychoanalysis... His soul rent in pieces with a view to reconstruction. The doctor says he is a tragedy: and his tragedy consists in the fact that he can't enjoy life with zest. I am probably responsible. I should have paired with him instead of hanging on to the elders. So he wilted pale, under a stone of vivacious brothers and sisters... For my part, I doubt if family life has all the power of evil attributed to it, or psychoanalysis of good.[22]

The same theme recurs in a letter to Vanessa, dated May 24, 1923: "Karin gave me an alarming account of Adrian's spiritual state. Apparently he has been broken down by the psychoanalysis (mentally) and has now to be put together.... I gather that his tragedy—as the dr. calls it—is all our doing. He was suppressed as a child."[23]

In 1924, Virginia began to comment on psychoanalysis in her role as publisher. On May 12, she wrote in her diary: "Dr. James Glover coming to discuss the P.S.S."[24] James Glover (1882-1926) was one of the earliest and most distinguished British psychoanalysts. He had come to see the Woolfs to make arrangements for the Hogarth Press to act as the official publishing house of the International Psycho-Analytical Library.

On September 22, 1924, she wrote to Roger Fry: "I have just finished your pamphlet [*The Artist and Psycho-Analysis*, published by the Hogarth Press in November 1924].... At the same time I am much annoyed about Clive."[25] The reference is to Clive Bell, whose article, "Dr. Freud on Art," appeared in the *Nation and Athenaeum* on September 6, 1922. At the end of this letter, Virginia returns to the subject of Freud and makes this cynical remark, so characteristic of her: "I'm rather alarmed at the productivity of the Hogarth Press this autumn—having laid out £800 in the work of Freud [*The Collected Papers*], which will sell they say because he has cancer."[26] Ten days later, while working on *Mrs. Dalloway*, she wrote to Molly MacCarthy:

We are publishing all Dr. Freud, and I glance at the proof and read how Mr. A. B. threw a bottle of red ink on to the sheets of his marriage bed to excuse his impotence to the housemaid, but threw it in the wrong place, which unhinged his wife's mind—and to this day she pours claret on the dinner table. We could all go on like that for hours; and yet these Germans think it proves something—besides their own gull-like imbecility.[27]

Virginia referred to Freud and psychoanalysts collectively as "these Germans." She knew better. She knew the difference between Austrians and Germans, and that Freud was a Jew. Oddly, she chose the word "glance" to describe her perusal of the proofs of Freud's *Collected Papers*. Perhaps she did only glance at the material, and that was enough to turn her off. Perhaps she read more deeply and did not want to dignify the author and his work by saying so. Astonishingly, a decade later, Virginia claimed that she was altogether unfamiliar with psychoanalysis. In 1932, replying to an inquiry by an American student, she wrote: *"I have not studied Dr. Freud or any psychoanalyst—indeed I think I have never read any of their books."*[28] Why did she lie about her familiarity with psychoanalysis?

On November 18, 1924, while preparing volumes I and II of Freud's *Collected Papers* for the printer, Virginia notes in her diary: "...doing up Freud."[29] This suggests she did more than "glance" at Freud's papers. From this date forward, Virginia's comments about Freud and psychoanalysis become increasingly disdainful. On May 22, 1927, in a letter to Vanessa, she paints a remarkable picture of psychoanalysis as a sort of spiritual rape: "I creep up and peer into the Stephens' dining room where any afternoon, in full daylight, is to be seen a woman in the last agony of despair, lying on a sofa, burying her face in the pillow while Adrian broods over her like a vulture, analyzing her soul."[30]

In the letter to the American student mentioned earlier, Virginia also makes a startling Freudian slip, which apparently has gone unnoticed. Presumably in reply to a query about the early publishing history of the Hogarth Press, she writes: "The titles of the two stories published by the Hogarth Press [in 1917] are *The Two Jews*, by my husband; and *The Mark on the Wall* by myself."[31] The title of Leonard's book was *The Three Jews*. What happened to the third Jew? Did Virginia "kill" him? She certainly forgot him. The editors of Virginia Woolf's *Letters* failed to append a footnote to the entry, noting the error. *Did they, too, overlook it? Or did they choose to not call attention to it?*

It is worth adding here that the most famous Bloomsburian, John Maynard Keynes, recognized very early that Freud was peddling ersatz religion, not medicine. "With religion dead and philosophy dry," he wrote in the *Manchester Guardian Commercial*, in January 1923, "the public run to witch-doctors. In cut and material our fig leaves have fallen out of fashion, and we find them neither comfortable nor becoming. Freud tells us to strip them off; Coué to wear two pairs."[32] With unerring perspicacity, Keynes saw through both the self-deluded postwar (World War I) political leaders who promised to make the world safe for democracy, and the self-deluded leaders of the then-emerging business of soul-doctoring who promised to cure man of the disease of the burden of living.[33]

Virginia had good reasons to fear and avoid psychoanalysts. The psychoanalytic relationship is intimate, in some ways more intimate than a sexual relationship. Its aim is to assist the "patient" to take a searching look at himself and stop deceiving himself. "Where id was, ego shall be," is the way Freud put it. I prefer to say that the aim of psychoanalysis is to make the inexplicit explicit, the metaphoric and indirect literal and direct. Doing so would have required exposing the lie that cemented the bond between Virginia and Leonard, that is, her playing the role of madwoman, and his playing the role of mental nurse. If Virginia feared that psychoanalysis might destabilize her marriage, she would have been right. Alix and James Strachey, who knew the Woolfs as well as anyone did, also thought so. According to Alix:

> [James] often wondered why Leonard did not persuade Virginia to see a psychoanalyst about her mental breakdowns. There were analysts with sufficient knowledge to understand her illness in those days. Although this knowledge was available, I did not agree with James that it would be of help to Virginia. Leonard, I think, might well have considered the proposition and *decided not to let her be psychoanalyzed...* Virginia's imagination, apart from her artistic creativeness, was so interwoven with her fantasies—and indeed with her madness—that if you had stopped the madness you might have stopped the creativeness too.... It may be preferable to be mad and be creative than to be treated by analysis and become ordinary.[34]

The Stracheys treat Virginia as if she were a child incapable of making decisions for herself, and seem utterly unaware of doing so. They talk about Virginia's conflicts and coping strategies as if they were diseases and assume that "treatment by analysis"—as if that were something other than conversation and self-conversation—could and might deprive her of her "creative powers." (Although the passage quoted does not refer to the potentially destabilizing effect of psychoanalysis on Virginia's marriage, I surmise that the thought occurred to both Alix and Virginia.)

5

After Virginia Woolf died, she quickly entered into the pantheon of feminist icons. She is the subject of numerous commentaries by feminists, some focusing specifically on her relationship to psycho-analysis. Most of the authors addressing the subject are uncritical of Woolf or Freud or both and seem unfamiliar with psychoanalysis as an historical-economic phenomenon and as a practice of "mental" healing.

Alma Halbert Bond's *Who Killed Virginia Woolf?* is amateurish. "Early in my professional career," she writes, "I dreamed that Freud and his colleagues were surrounded by a great magnetic force which lifted me off the ground until I was as tall as they. Psychoanalysis has indeed lifted me to greater heights than I could ever have dreamed of, for instance to writing the psychobiography of Virginia Woolf."[35]

Couched in convoluted, pretentious prose, the thesis of Elizabeth Abel's *Virginia Woolf and the Fictions of Psychoanalysis* is confused and self-contradictory. She states: "[Virginia Woolf's] stories echo and rewrite the developmental *fictions of psychoanalysis....* The ques-tion of Woolf's relation to psychoanalysis has usually been posed as either a question of her response to Freud or of her anticipation of a mother-based theory."[36] Mother-based theory of *what*? Mental ill-ness? In both the title and the text of her book, Abel refers to the *fictions of psychoanalysis.*

Her book, Abel explains, "examines and contextualizes this ex-change within the historical moment Woolf shared with Sigmund Freud and Melanie Klein.... Woolf's fiction...de-authorizes psycho-analysis, clarifying the narrative choices it makes, disclosing its fictionality."[37] The authority, if any, of psychoanalysis does not de-pend on Virginia Woolf's novels. If psychoanalytic accounts are fic-tions, there is nothing to fictionalize. The fictionality of psychoanaly-sis was revealed long before Abel was born.[38]

The authoritative *Cambridge Companion to Virginia Woolf*, ed-ited by Sue Roe and Susan Sellers, contains a chapter by Nicole Ward Jouve, a French feminist writer, promisingly titled, "Virginia Woolf and psychoanalysis."[39] It's a disappointment. Jouve writes: "Psychoanalysis is the science and clinical practice that was born from Freud's discovery of the unconscious...Freud's invention of the 'talking cure' placed language firmly at the center of its theory and practice.... It has led to new ways of looking at art, new ways of reading texts, literature in particular."[40] Psychoanalysis is not a science, there is nothing "clinical" (medical) about it, and "the unconscious" is a concept or construct, not a thing to be "discovered."

Jouve puts words and sentences on paper that tell us nothing: "Woolf herself suffered from bouts of insanity. Yet psychoanalysis does not seem to have been considered as a possible cure, least of all by herself: might it have helped?"[41] She does not answer the question. She changes the subject and writes about mental illness as if it were an illness like melanoma: "There are divergent versions of the severity, frequency, and nature of Woolf's mental illness, and even of what the diagnosis should be: manic depression? Cyclothymia (i.e., periodic breakdowns interspersed by long periods of sanity)? Hysteria? Schizophrenia?... Hermione Lee states: 'Virginia was a sane woman who had an illness.... Her illness is attributable to genetic, environmental, and biological factors.'"[42] Like Lee, Jouve likes the idea that Virginia was wholly innocent of her misbehavior while insane. She did not kill herself. Her genes, environment, "biological factors," in short, mental illness, killed her.

Jouve writes to impress, not to inform. Rhetorically, she asks: "Is it the case that such understandings were in the air anyway, that a novelist like Woolf and a scientist like Freud were at the same time and with different means exploring the same psychic realities? Should a fluid notion of intertextuality replace that of influence?"[43] With "psychic realities" and "a fluid notion of intertextuality," we enter the land of Alice-in-Wonderland deconstructionism. The eye glazes over. Or else it glows with the flame of the faith of secular gullibility.

Is this the best account of the connections between Virginia Woolf and psychoanalysis that the editors of *The Cambridge Companion to Virginia Woolf* can provide?

There is not much of value in the voluminous literature on the connections between psychoanalysis and Virginia Woolf's life and work, as my brief review of illustrative examples shows. An exception of sort is the document, "Bloomsbury and Psychoanalysis: An Exhibition of Documents from the Archives of the British Psychoanalytical Society," compiled by Polly Rossdale and Ken Robinson.[44] Abstaining from analytical commentary, the compilers present a wealth of valuable information about the personal connections between the Bloomsbury group and the individuals who formed the nucleus of psychoanalysis in England.

6

Was Virginia wise to avoid seeking psychoanalytic help? The answer depends on the respondent's opinion of Virginia Woolf, Sigmund Freud, and psychoanalysis. I believe Virginia was wise to avoid becoming a psychoanalytic patient, especially Freud's patient. My reason for this judgment rests partly on what I believe Virginia wanted out of life, and partly on my understanding of the nature of Freud's interest in art, artists, and psychoanalysis.

In his essay on the "History of the Psycho-Analytic Movement," Freud defines psychoanalysis as a method for "investigating the life of the mind."[45] This definition is an invitation to epistemological and logical mischief. It implies that just as plants, animals, and humans have lives, so also do minds. We may dismiss this view as nonsense or consider it a classic case of a category error. This definition also identifies psychoanalysis as a method or "instrument." The metaphor is Freud's.[46] As the microscope is useful for investigating microbes, so psychoanalysis is useful for investigating the "mind." That sounds like a good thing for the investigator, who, especially if he is among the pioneers in the use of the instrument, is likely to become famous for seeing things no one else had seen before. Yet, elsewhere, Freud explicitly rejects the notion that the analyst uses an instrument: "Nothing takes place between them [analyst and analysand] except that they talk to each other. The analyst makes use of no instruments—not even for examining the patient— nor does he prescribe any medicines."[47]

Thus, one of the problems with "having a method for investigating the mind" is that, as I have noted, the mind is an abstract idea, not a physical object. Investigating a person's mind is not like investigating his liver; it is like investigating, say, his imagination.[48] Furthermore, if we talk about a psychoanalyst's investigating his patient's mind, we must ask: What would such an investigation, if successful, be good for? Whom would it benefit? In the hard sciences, investigation helps the investigator, not the investigated. Investigating the malaria parasite helps the microbiologist, the physician, and the malaria patient, not the pathogenic microorganism. *Mutatis mutandis*, psychoanalysis helps the psychoanalyst: It enriches his "mind" and wallet. What, if anything, does it do for the patient? It is a matter of fact, not logic, whether such an "investigation" helps him, harms him, or is indifferent for his well being. To be sure, if by psychoanalysis we mean a simultaneous investigation of the patient by the analyst and a self-investigation by the patient, then the patient may also benefit.[49]

Clearly, psychoanalysis is attractive for the psychoanalyst. He can make use of his powerful "instrument," gain knowledge thereby, and get paid in the bargain. There is nothing in psychoanalysis that is clearly beneficial for the would-be patient. In this respect, too, psychoanalysis differs from medical treatment, which is expected to benefit the patient, not the doctor. To make the prospect of being a psychoanalytic patient even less attractive, especially for someone like Virginia Woolf, Freud emphasized that the analytic situation is one "in which there is a superior and a subordinate."[50] It is clear which position he had in mind for the patient.

Freud's specification that psychoanalysis "is not suited...for polemical use" presents still more problems.[51] The assertion is not true. Freud himself never tired of using psychoanalysis polemically, for example as a weapon against living disloyal disciples like Adler and Jung, as well as against famous dead persons like Leonardo da Vinci and Woodrow Wilson.

Finally, there is Freud's troubling double-talk about confidentiality in the analytic situation. On the one hand, he explains: "With the neurotics, then, we make our pact: complete candor on one side and strict discretion on the other."[52] But he also states: "I make use of his [patient's] communication without asking his consent, since I cannot allow that a psycho-analytic technique has any right to claim the protection of medical discretion."[53]

Freud was not particularly interested in helping his patients. He did that for a living. His heart lay in the advancement of his "cause" by the recruitment of disciples, and in psychoanalysis as a method for penetrating into the "secrets" of artists and for exposing "fakes." When his colleague, Theodor Reik, compared him to Sherlock Holmes, Freud responded by acknowledging that he also saw himself as a sleuth and identified himself especially with Giovanni Morelli, a nineteenth-century art scholar famous for his skill in "detecting fakes."[54] Freud also compared psychoanalytic treatment to a detective's investigating a crime and finding the criminal: He wrote: "I must draw an analogy between the criminal and the hysteric. In both we are concerned with a secret, with something hidden."[55] The analogy between the psychoanalyst and the detective is part of the larger theme of Freud's metaphors, masterfully explored by Stanley

Edgar Hyman in *The Tangled Bank*. Hyman calls attention to the violent imagery of many of Freud's metaphors, such as his description of the psychoanalyst's method for making a diagnosis, which Freud describes as follows:

> We are in fact buying a pig in a poke. The patient brings along indefinite general ailments which do not admit of a conclusive diagnosis.... Our diagnoses are very often made only after the event. They resemble the Scottish King's test for identifying witches that I read about in Victor Hugo. This king declared that he was in possession of an infallible method of recognizing a witch. He had the woman stewed in a cauldron of boiling water and then tasted the broth. Afterwards he was able to say: "That was a witch," or "No, that was not one." It is the same with us, *except that we are the sufferers*.[56]

The final flourish is vintage Freud, denying that he is the victimizer, declaring himself the victim. The metaphor is characteristic of Freud's style and epitomizes everything Virginia Woolf scorned and fought against her whole life: the woman represented as witch; the male-female relationship represented as a king boiling and eating women; a doctor offering this scenario as a metaphor for diagnosing mental illness. Perhaps it is not entirely coincidental that Virginia should have written: "When, however, one reads of a witch being ducked, of a woman possessed by devils...then I think we are on the track of a lost novelist."[57] Even Hilda Doolittle (1886-1961)—an expatriate American writer, patient, and admirer of Freud—characterized him as a "terribly frightening old man."[58]

Freud liked to think of himself, and wanted others to think of him, as an angry man. In 1931, a group of analysts commissioned the subsequently world-famous Yugoslav-born sculptor Oscar Nemon (1906-1985) to make a bust of the Master for his seventy-fifth birthday. Heinrich Meng, who received one of the copies, provided the following revealing glimpse into what happened: "Nemon did not allow Freud to look at his work before it was finished, but when the bust was almost finished he showed it to Freud's housekeeper, who said, 'The Professor looks too angry with humanity.' When the statue was finished, Freud looked at it and remarked, 'I am glad you put in enough anger.'"[59] We have encountered this image of the angry Jew before in this essay, in Thoby Stephen's explanation of Leonard Woolf's tremor. Leonard trembled, Thoby told Virginia, because "he so despised the whole human race." Probably one angry Jew was enough for Virginia.

5

"A screwed up shrunk very old man"

1

Freud was keenly interested in art, artists, and famous people in general; he wrote about Leonardo da Vinci, Michelangelo, Shakespeare, Dostoyevsky, and Woodrow Wilson. "There is a special charm," he remarked, "in studying the psychic lives of human beings in the distinguished individual."[1] What did Freud mean by qualifying "lives" with "psychic" (*psychisch*)?

When Freud declares his interest in the "psychic lives" of famous persons, he is telling us that he proposes to use their psyches as the pathologist uses cadavers: After he dissects them with his psychoanalytic scalpel, they will yield their pathological secrets to him. Freud is not interested in peoples' lives the way an ordinary person or a biographer or a novelist is. Nor is he interested in how people see their own lives. Instead, his interest in famous people is like the forensic pathologist's interest in the corpses of persons who die under mysterious circumstances. He wants to cut them open with his scalpel to uncover their "secrets."

Indeed, Stefan Zweig, the author of an admiring mini-biography of Freud, uses the scalpel metaphor to characterize Freud's analytic "method": "If Nietzsche philosophizes with a hammer, Freud philosophizes with a scalpel; and neither of these implements would be of any value in hands too gentle, too considerate, to make good use of them."[2]

The view that Freud's method of analyzing patients, religion, art, and famous people was invasive and destructive, resembling rape, is supported by another metaphor, dear to Freud's own heart, that of the detective ferreting out a secret. With this metaphor-weapon in hand, Freud commits a kind of moral suicide.

Cui bono? Who benefits from the detective's detection of a secret? Assuredly, not the criminal hiding the secret. The detective's job is to harm, not help, the criminal; in the process, he also helps himself and the society he protects from criminals. We see here how readily, in fact eagerly, Freud fell into the traditional role of the psychiatrist. After the psychoanalytic dissection is completed and the "mysterious core" of the subject's "psyche" has been successfully "penetrated," Freud considers the problem "solved," the psychoanalytically demystified object/subject catalogued and displayed with the discoverer's other trophies.

Clearly, Freud was interested in famous artists because they were famous, not because they were artists. Thomas Mann, unfailingly deferential toward Freud, recognized this. In 1925, he wrote: "As an artist, I have to confess, however, that I am not at all satisfied with Freudian ideas; rather, I feel disquieted and reduced by them. The artist is being x-rayed by Freud's ideas to the point where *it violates the secret of his creative art*."[3] And in 1930, in a letter to Freud, Mann reproached him for it: "You love writers? Probably mainly as objects of your research."[4]

Long before analysts were called "shrinks," Mann called attention to the fact that psychoanalysis—like many other ostensibly liberating enterprises—is a knife that cuts both ways. Education may be used to enlighten or to indoctrinate; medicine, to cure or to kill; psychoanalysis, to expand and enrich the mind or to shrink and impoverish it.

2

One of the clearest descriptions of the destructive, penetrative, rape-like quality of what Freud meant by explaining something psychoanalytically appears in his essay titled "The Moses of Michelangelo,"[5] a piece he published anonymously, accompanied with a lie: An "explanatory note" represented the writer as an "anonymous author whose mode of thought has in point of fact a certain resemblance to the methodology of psychoanalysis." Freud waited ten years before revealing that he was the author and never explained why he had lied about it.

Freud acknowledged that he was not interested in art for art's sake. He was interested in art only as a sign or symptom pointing to something more interesting and important for him, what he called the "secret" of the artistic "product":

I have often observed that the subject matter of works of art has a stronger attraction for me than their formal or technical qualities.... I am unable rightly to appreciate many of the methods used and the effects obtained in art.... Nevertheless, works of art do exercise a powerful effect on me, especially those of literature and sculpture, less often of painting. This has occasioned me, when I have been contemplating things, to spend a long time before trying to apprehend them *in my own way*, i.e., to explain to myself what their effect is due to. Whenever I cannot do this, *as for instance with music*, I am almost incapable of obtaining any pleasure. Some rationalistic, or perhaps analytic, turn of mind in me *rebels against being moved* by a thing without knowing why I am thus affected and what it is that affects me.[6]

The similarity between Freud's attitude toward art and Virginia's toward sex is striking: Neither wants to be affected/penetrated by something that he/she considers alien and does not control, something that might move or excite him/her. We call such a woman sexually frigid. Freud was artistically frigid. Virginia avoids sex or must experience it under her own control and on her own terms (perhaps by masturbation). Freud avoids art (as art) or must experience it under his own control and on his own terms by transforming it into a "product" that he can "analyze." Each refracts powerful human experiences through her or his own personal prejudices that, however, tap deep currents in their cultures. Unable and unwilling to see sexual activity as a source of intimacy and joy, Virginia—the Puritan—is interested in it only as defilement and dirt. Unable and unwilling to see artistic and religious activity as a source of beauty and joy, Freud—the man of the Enlightenment—is interested in it only as insanity and illusion. And so he justifies his "analysis" of art by postulating a problem where, in fact, there is none.

The more Freud writes about art and artists, the more clearly he reveals his destructive attitude toward both. He complains that different lovers of art say different things about why they admire the statue, but "none of them says anything that *solves the problem* for the unpretending admirer."[7] What problem? Freud plants a secret on the corpse and, after an elaborately staged psychoanalytic dissection of it, he triumphantly produces it: "In my opinion, what grips us so powerfully can only be the artists' *intention*.... But why should the artist's intention not be capable of being communicated and comprehended in *words*, like any other fact of mental life? Perhaps where great works of art are concerned, this would never be possible *without the application of psychoanalysis*. The *product itself* after all must admit of such an analysis."[8]

This is sheer chutzpah. The world's great works of art, Freud implies, have somehow remained unfinished throughout the ages, awaiting their completion through Freudian psychoanalysis. Freud's premise—that all "facts of mental life" (whatever that pretentious phrase means) must be expressible in words—is nonsense. Nonverbal expressions—not only those mentioned by Freud but also other forms, such as dance and, perhaps most importantly, silence itself—are as much a part of the cultural heritage and life of mankind as are words. Freud knew this. But since those "products" could not be subjected to his "analytic method," he ignored them, concentrating on those art forms that could, in principle at least, be degraded into "materials" subject to psychoanalytic interpretation. Freud acknowledged that such interpretation was his ultimate aim: "To discover the [artist's] intention...I must first find out the meaning and content of what is represented in his work; *I must, in other words, be able to interpret it.*"[9]

Freud recognized that critics might consider his "psychoanalytic interpretation" of art as an act of hostility or violence against the artist and his work, and so disavowed having such motives: "Investigations of this kind [that is, psychoanalytic pathographies] are not intended to explain an author's genius..."[10] If they are not intended to do that, what are they intended to do? Elsewhere he states: "I even venture to hope that the effect of the work will undergo no diminution after we have succeeded in thus analyzing it.... When psychiatric [*seelenärztliche*] research, normally content to draw on frailer men for its material, approaches one who is among the greatest of the human race, it is not doing so for reasons so frequently ascribed to it by laymen. [Quoting Schiller:] 'To blacken the radiant and drag the sublime into the dust' is no part of its purpose."[11] I submit that Freud and his followers are guilty of "psychoanalyzing" great artists and famous people precisely in order to blacken their names. Freud's essays on famous artists and his book on Woodrow Wilson are ample proof of the validity of this charge.[12]

When Freud turns to illustrating the process of psychoanalyzing a great work of art, his competitiveness with its creator and his desire to destroy the art and triumph over the artist are plain. In his essay on Leonardo da Vinci, after stating his disclaimer, Freud continues: "But it [psychoanalysis] cannot help finding worthy of understanding everything that can be recognized in those illustrious models, and it believes there is no one so great as to be disgraced by being subject to the laws which govern both normal and pathological activity with equal cogency."[13] Note that Freud elevates his "laws" to the level of natural laws, on a par with the laws governing, say, the movement of the planets. In human affairs, there are no such laws.

A few pages later, Freud lets himself go so far as to declare: "The slowness which had all along been conspicuous in Leonardo's work is seen to be a *symptom* of this *inhibition* and to be the forerunner of his subsequent withdrawal from painting. It was this too which determined the fate of the Last Supper—a fate that was not undeserved."[14] Who is Freud to judge how rapidly Leonardo da Vinci should paint? To my knowledge, neither Freud nor his admirers have ever explained, or even recognized, his glee about the deterioration of Leonardo's immortal fresco, a fate attributable to the nature of the wall on which it was painted and the atmosphere to which it was exposed, not the slowness of his work.

Freud trawls for every scrap of information about Leonardo, only to "interpret" it as a "symptom" of his homosexuality: "He was gentle and kindly to everyone; he declined, it is said, to eat meat, since he did not think it justifiable to deprive animals of their lives; and he took particular pleasure in buying birds in the market and setting them free. He condemned war and bloodshed."[15] All of this shows that Leonardo was an effeminate homosexual?

Two pages later, we read: "It is doubtful whether Leonardo ever embraced a woman in passion.... While he was still an apprentice, living in the house of his master Verrocchio, a charge of forbidden homosexual practices was brought against him, along with some other young people, which ended in his acquittal."[16] The court might have acquitted Leonardo. Freud didn't. His whole essay is devoted to proving that Leonardo was a homosexual, his main evidence for it based, ironically, on a mistranslation of the word "kite" as "vulture."[17] "If we examine with the eyes of a psycho-analyst," Freud pontificates, "Leonardo's fantasy of a vulture, it does not appear strange for long."[18] But there was no vulture; Leonardo never mentioned a vulture. In the end, Freud shows his hand: "What decides whether we describe someone as an invert [homosexual] is not his actual behavior, but his emotional attitude."[19] This method for judging character resembles the Catholic inquisitorial standard for judging "thought crimes" too closely for comfort.

Shakespeare, too, was one of Freud's targets. "Let us consider"—he writes in his "Moses" essay, pretending he is not the writer—

"Shakespeare's masterpiece *Hamlet*, a play now over three centuries old. I have followed the literature of psychoanalysis closely, and I accept its claim that it was not until the material of the tragedy had been traced back by psychoanalysis to the Oedipus theme that the *mystery of its effect* was at last explained."[20] Nothing means what it means. It means only what Freud says it means. Freud's psychoanalytic reconstruction prefigures Derrida's nihilistic de-construction.

Freud's language is at once pompous and deceptive. It is not he who self-interestedly advances a claim; it is the disinterested science of psychoanalysis that does so. The "real" effect of *Hamlet* lies not in Shakespeare's art but in Freud's explanation of the "mystery" of its effect. Freud is competing with Shakespeare and tries to best him. Perhaps this is why he lied about the provenance of this essay: He could compare himself with Shakespeare without being accused of doing so. Freud's essay on Woodrow Wilson is a "smoking gun," proving beyond reasonable doubt that he was happy to use the "psychoanalytic method" as a rhetorical weapon.[21]

Many observers of Freud's writings on art have noted that there was more to this enterprise than Freud acknowledged. The German philosopher of art Ludwig Marcuse suggests that Freud's preoccupation with and search for the "content" of works of art accounts for his inability to enjoy music, and much else besides: "Freud deceived himself when he said that *only* in relation to music was he almost incapable of enjoyment. However, his general incapacity was brought out particularly clearly by music, because in general it lacks...what Freud calls *content*.... But Freud's equation of the pleasure of *understanding* a work of art with *enjoyment* of art simply shows how little he knew of this specific enjoyment."[22] Marcuse was on to Freud's competitive-destructiveness, but was not interested in this subject and did not pursue it.

The results of Freud's "psychoanalytic pathographies" were foreordained and were always the same. On one side, the subject, a "distinguished individual" who, seen in the light of the higher "truth" of psychoanalysis, is "really" a pathetic mental case, riddled with psychopathological symptoms, incapable of recognizing, much less controlling, his unconscious drives or impulses. On the other side, the master interpreter of human behavior, armed with the tools of the science of psychoanalysis, unmasks and reveals the "truth" about art, religion, psychic life, and, of course, madness. Stefan Zweig sensed this arbitrary, autocratic quality of Freud's mind but, restrained by his admiration of the Master, could state it only obliquely: "Unless Freud understands a thing promptly and unconditionally, it remains inaccessible to him; and no one can explain anything to him unless, of his own self, he can grasp it without reserve. He is thus unfailingly autocratic and intransigent."[23]

In my view, Freud's pervasive anger toward the world rendered his character—as it renders that of every overzealous "reformer"—deficient in what I call basic decency. Freud recognized that his probing of the innermost recesses of a person's soul was similar to the priest's probing of the innermost recesses of the penitent's soul in the confessional, and he was aware that the probity of such a method is contingent on the inviolable confidentiality of the relationship. Nevertheless, he disrespected this stricture in psychoanalysis proper, and brazenly rejected it when he applied his method to historical figures.

Freud rejected, or was incapable of maintaining, the kind of discretion upon which the very method of "treatment" associated with his name depends. He rationalized this choice (or failing) as fearless truth-telling. But judging people on the basis of motives attributed to them by the psychoanalyst, and defining the judgment as "fact" arrived at by the "scientific method of psychoanalysis"—rather than judging them on the basis of their overt behavior, as the tradition of English law teaches—is not truth-telling. It is the very opposite of truth-telling.

Is psychoanalysis, then—especially in Freud's hands—a method of unmasking the patient's embarrassing secrets for the benefit of the psychoanalyst, or a method of enriching the client's self-understanding and enhancing his well being by augmenting his responsibility and liberty? If the answer is that psychoanalysis is a tool for benefiting only the analyst, then the Austrian satirist Karl Kraus was right when he pronounced it "the disease of which it pretends to be the cure."

And René Laforgue, one of the pioneer French psychoanalysts, was also right when he declared that psychoanalysis was "a religion to which it is forbidden to give its true name."[24]

Otto Rank, too, was right when he finally concluded that "analysis has become the worst enemy of the soul."[25]

And Virginia Woolf, too, was right that it was better to be Freud's publisher than his patient.

3

Virginia Woolf and Sigmund Freud differed in gender, social background, profession, and lifestyle. However, both were gifted writers; both were preoccupied, to the exclusion of much else in their lives, with madness; and each played the roles of both "mental patient" and "analyst-therapist." Virginia's main goal in life, like Freud's, was to become famous: Virginia wanted to be a famous writer; Freud, a famous discoverer.

Virginia became a famous writer whose principal subject was her own life. Freud became a famous "doctor" as well as his most intensively studied "patient." Both were grand maskers of themselves, and unmaskers of others. Virginia Woolf tamed conflict as fiction; Freud, as psychopathology. Virginia recognized, as Freud did also, that the analyst and the novelist are competitors: Each endeavors to portray, *with words*, an existentially faithful understanding of human behavior, feelings, and relationships. Freud was honored as a great writer with a Goethe Prize, not as a great medical discoverer with a Nobel Prize.

Virginia Woolf and Sigmund Freud both created their own publishing houses, an unusual enterprise for either writer or doctor. Both assumed and played the twin roles of writer and publisher of their own texts, a role befitting the religious or political propagandist, rather than the novelist or therapist. Each was a devout atheist who, nevertheless, strongly identified with her or his own "race," class, and cultural heritage. Both were arrogant snobs, a trait displayed by disdain toward "outsiders," Virginia toward Jews, Freud toward gentiles. Finally, both Woolf and Freud were exceedingly "narcissistic." When the Woolfs visited Freud in London near the end of his life, Freud presented Virginia with a symbolically suggestive gift. And therein lies a tale worth telling.

In the years between the world wars, Giovanni Papini (1881-1956) was a well-known Italian writer, poet, critic, and a pioneer of the modern literary form of fiction as "fact."[26] He wrote widely read imagined interviews with famous people, among them one with Freud.[27]

In the spring of 1933, according to the story, Papini comes across an old Greek statuette of Narcissus. Familiar with Freud's interest in such antiques, Papini sends it to him, accompanied by a letter paying homage to the "discoverer of Narcissism" on his recently celebrated seventy-seventh birthday. Freud invites Papini to visit him.

Papini travels to Vienna and writes an essay about their imagined conversation. It was published, in an English translation, in the British magazine *Colosseum* in 1934.

There is no evidence that the interview ever took place. However, some Freud scholars mistook, and continue to mistake, Papini's account for a real event. Still, the "interview" remains of interest because it articulates with especial clarity and force "Freud's" view of the nonmedical—one might say "antipsychiatric"—character of psychoanalysis.

Freud greets Papini warmly and expresses delight that Papini is "neither a patient, nor colleague, nor a disciple, nor a relative...at last I can speak freely to you."[28] Freud begins by complaining:

> Everybody thinks that I stand by the scientific character of my work... This is a terrible error that has prevailed for years and that I have been unable to set right.... I am really by nature an artist. Ever since childhood, my secret hero has been Goethe. I would have liked to become a poet, and my whole life long I've wanted to write novels. But...my family was poor, and poetry, on the testimony of the most celebrated contemporaries, brought in little... Moreover, I was a Jew...[in] an anti-Semite monarchy. Heine's exile and wretched end discouraged me.[29]

Freud, according to Papini's fictitious but realistic interview, felt handicapped and stigmatized because he was a Jew. Virginia Woolf felt this way because she was a woman. Both sought their salvation in the Word, in self-affirmation through literature. Virginia Woolf was a professional writer. Freud was a professional doctor, but that role was a pretense: "A man of letters by instinct, though a doctor by necessity, I conceived the idea of changing over a branch of medicine—psychiatry—into literature. Though I have the appearance of a scientist, I was and am a poet and novelist. Psychoanalysis is no more than the interpretation of a literary vocation in terms of psychology and pathology."[30] Many students of psychoanalysis, myself included, have said this. Here, Papini put the interpretation directly into Freud's mouth. Papini went further. Freud (supposedly) told Papini that his crediting the discovery of catharsis to Breuer was a tactic, a ruse to give it a medical gloss. In truth, he got the idea from Goethe, Hugo, and Zola:

> [T]he first impulse which led to the discovery of my method came to me from my beloved Goethe. As you must know, he wrote *Werther* to free himself from the morbid oppression of a sorrow: for him literature meant a *catharsis*.

And in what consists my method of curing hysteria save in making the patient tell everything to free him from obsession? I did no more than force my patients to act like Goethe. Confession is liberation and that is cure. The Catholics knew it for centuries, but Victor Hugo had taught me that the poet too is a priest: and thus I boldly substituted myself for the confessor. The first step was taken.[31]

Papini's presentation was credible; indeed, in 1934, it was commonplace. Today—when psychoanalysis is accepted as a part of psychiatry, and when health insurance programs pay for psychoanalytic "treatment"—it is unalloyed heresy. But Freud was not yet finished with *his* "confession":

I very soon realized that the confessions of my patients formed a precious selection of "human documents." That is to say, I carried out the same plan as Zola. He turned these documents into novels—I was constrained to keep them to myself. Then my attention was drawn to the similarity between dreams and works of art and the importance of the language of symbols... *Psychoanalysis was born—not as they say through the suggestions of Breuer but as a result of the scientific transposition of the literary schools I like best.*[32]

Breuer, psychiatry, diagnosis, illness—the whole medical edifice of psychoanalytic theory—all is a disguise, *a mask to conceal that psychoanalysis is the existential-literary interpretation of the human condition.*
Virginia hid her true self behind a mask of mental illness or in the persona of a fictional figure. Freud hid his true self behind a mask of dream interpretation and a novel form of "mental healing." The repressed, true self, however, returns and finds ways of reasserting itself. Cleverly, Papini pretended that Freud was "confessing" to him the inadmissible truth about psychoanalysis, a truth at which Freud himself often hinted:

My soul, by its constitution, leans towards the essay, the paradox, the dramatic, and has nothing of the pedantic technical stiffness which belongs to the true man of science... My books, in fact, more resemble works of imagination than treatises on pathology... I have been able to win my destiny in an indirect way, and have attained my dream: to remain a man of letters, though still in appearance a doctor.[33]

This interpretation prefigures Stanley Edgar Hyman's fine study of Freud as an imaginative writer, much as Papini's gift to Freud prefigures Freud's gift to Virginia. At the end of the interview, Freud tells Papini that "Nobody has noticed this open secret [that he is a writer disguised as a doctor] and I would have revealed it to no one if you had not had the splendid idea of presenting me with a statue of Narcissus."[34]

In the fall of 1938, Freud fled Vienna and settled, for the few remaining months of his life, in London. In January 1939 Virginia and Leonard Woolf visited him in his home in Hampstead. Freud, reserved but cordial, presented Virginia with a single narcissus. Virginia reciprocated by pronouncing Freud "a screwed up shrunk very old man."[35]

Virginia Woolf was then a very screwed up prematurely old woman. She survived Freud by only two years.

6

"He will go on, better without me"

Sir Leslie Stephen was a devout atheist. His views on suicide, to which Virginia never referred, may have provided a moral rationale for her conviction that she had a right to kill herself, that by committing suicide she was doing good, not evil.

In 1882, the year of Virginia's birth, Leslie Stephen published one of his major works, revealingly titled *The Science of Ethics*. Against the mainstream of official Victorian thought, yet in a style deeply characteristic of his age and class, Stephen presented a passionate argument for the morality of suicide. He wrote:

> If, now, we suppose that a man, knowing that life meant for him nothing but agony, and that moreover his life could not serve others, and was only going to give useless pain to his attendants, and perhaps involve the sacrifice of health to his wife and children, should commit suicide, what ought we to think of him? He would, no doubt, be breaking the accepted moral code; but why should he not break it?... May we not say that he is acting on a superior moral principle, and that because he is clearly diminishing the sum of human misery?... The conduct may spring either from cowardice or from a loftier motive than the ordinary, and the merit of the action is therefore not determinable; but, assuming the loftier motive, I can see no ground for disapproving that action which flows from it.[1]

Leslie Stephen did not kill himself. He chose to die a lingering and painful death from cancer.

2

Following the Nazi occupation of France in 1940, the Woolfs and many of their friends feared for their lives in case of a successful German invasion of England. They made preparations to commit

81

suicide. Some thirty years later, Leonard looked back at those days and wrote: "Adrian told us that he would commit suicide rather than fall into German hands, and that he had provided himself with means of doing so; he offered Virginia and me...a portion of this protective poison. I gather from Harold Nicolson's memoirs that he and Vita [Sackville-West] provided themselves with a similar 'bare bodkin'... [here] were five ordinary intelligent people in England, coolly and prudently supplying themselves with means for committing suicide."[2]

The drug was morphine, a substance many famous people used to kill themselves when threatened with capture by the Nazis. Note that the people who spent decades trying to protect Virginia from suicide were now willing to supply her with the means for doing so easily and painlessly; and that the people who, when Virginia feared life without her mother, considered suicide to be irrational, a manifestation of madness, regarded it, when they feared life under Nazi rule, rational, a manifestation of sanity.

With psychiatry as his religion, Leonard was ready to attribute madness to almost any behavior of which he disapproved—from Virginia's suicide to Hitler's politics. Invariably, he referred to Hitler as a madman and to Nazism as a form of insanity: "Europeans had slipped into the hands of a sadistic madman"; "[T]he Germans were now infected with his insanity"; "There was something insane in Hitler's genocide"; "[T]his sadistic nightmare of an insane megalomaniac"; "[I]nfected with Hitler's sadistic insanity."[3] It did not seem to occur to Leonard that if he used the idea of insanity to explain Hitler's beliefs and policies *as well as* Virginia Woolf's creativity and suicide, he explained nothing. According to Leonard:

> Death was always very near the surface of Virginia's mind, the contemplation of death. It was part of the deep imbalance of her mind. She was "half in love with easeful Death.".... I hardly ever even thought of death.... It is in part due perhaps to the Jewish tradition.... Virginia's attitude to death was very different. It was always present to her. The fact that she had twice tried to commit suicide...meant that death was never far from her thoughts.[4]

Note that Leonard regarded Virginia's "contemplation of death," as "part of the deep imbalance of her mind." Mental health was his religion. In that faith, thinking about dying is "suicidal ideation," a symptom of severe mental illness.[5] Alas, if only life were that simple.

Ironically, it was Leonard, not Virginia, who, at that time, was preoccupied with the idea of suicide. He writes: "We agreed that, if the time came, there would be no point in waiting; we would shut the garage door and commit suicide." Once again, Leonard missed the mark. Virginia didn't like the idea: "I don't want the garage to see the end of me."[6]

The Germans invaded France in May 1940. Virginia killed herself on March 28, 1941. Less than eleven months had elapsed since Adrian had provided the Woolfs with lethal quantities of morphine to prevent Nazi capture. Was she in possession of that drug then, or ever? If so, why did she not use it? Or was the morphine always in Leonard's hands? In my extensive reading about these events, I have found no information regarding these questions. Whatever the answers, I consider Virginia's preparation for her self-determined death to be just as coolly and prudently calculated as Adrian's and Leonard's had been a few months earlier.

3

Leonard was right when he observed that the idea of suicide was never far from Virginia's mind. When she was twenty-two, she jumped from a low window without sustaining any injury. This "hysterical" (in the old-fashioned sense) act—a suicidal gesture, at worst— was interpreted as a suicide attempt. After marrying Leonard, Virginia made a more serious attempt at suicide when she overdosed on sleeping pills, and thereafter kept him perpetually terrorized with the threat that she would kill herself. Finally, he gave up the charade of caring, and she drowned herself.

In October 1930, in a letter to Ethel Smyth, Virginia, like her father, pondered the moral legitimacy of suicide:

> By the way, what are the arguments against suicide? You know what a flibbertigibbet I am: well there suddenly comes in a thunder clap a sense of the complete uselessness of my life. It's like suddenly running one's head against a wall at the end of a blind alley. Now what are the arguments against that sense—"Oh it would be better to end it"? I need not say that I have no sort of intention of taking any steps: I simply want to know...what are the arguments against it?[7]

Here Virginia might have cited her father's meditations on suicide in *The Science of Ethics*. But she didn't. Had she read the book?

In March 1931, she confided to Smyth: "Why did I feel violent after the party? It would be amusing to see how far you can make out, with your insight, the various states of mind which led me, on coming home, to say to L:—'If you weren't here, I should kill my-self—so much do I suffer.'"[8] A few days later, after hearing Beatrice Webb discuss suicide, she wrote to her: "I wanted to tell you but was too shy, how much I was pleased by your views upon the possible justification of suicide. Having made the attempt myself, from the best of motives as I thought—not to be a burden on my husband—the con-ventional accusation of cowardice and sin has always rather rankled."[9]

In 1941, Virginia was nearing sixty. The war was going badly. The words she wrote in *Mrs. Dalloway* may have echoed in her ears: "*She* could not grow old and have no children! She was very lonely, she was very unhappy!"[10] The Woolfs' house in Mecklenburg Square had been heavily damaged by bombs. Virginia may have sensed that Leonard, preoccupied with the dire political situation in Europe, was getting tired of her. Perhaps she was getting tired of writing. In December 1940, Virginia wrote Octavia Wilberforce, a general prac-titioner, Sussex neighbor, and the last doctor to see Virginia: "I've lost all power over words, can't do a thing with them."[11]

In February 1941, the writer Elizabeth Bowen visited Virginia and "found no sign of illness." Some days before March 18, Virginia "returned from a walk soaking wet, saying that she had fallen."[12] It is likely that she had tried to drown herself in the river Ouse, near her Sussex home, but changed her mind. Leonard made no attempt to control her by psychiatric intervention. Finally, on March 28, Vir-ginia succeeded in killing herself. She had put stones in the pocket of her coat to weigh down her body and walked into the river Ouse. Twenty days later, her body was recovered. An inquest was held, and the verdict was: "Suicide while the balance of her mind was disturbed." Her body was cremated.

Killing herself with morphine would have been easier on Virginia as well as on Leonard. She dramatized herself to the end. She left two suicide notes to Leonard, and one to Vanessa. I reproduce all three below, in that order.

Dearest, I feel certain I am going mad again. I feel we can't go through another of those terrible times. And I shan't recover this time. I begin to hear voices, and I can't concentrate. So I am doing what seems the best thing to do. You have given me the greatest possible happiness. You have been in every way all that anyone could be. *I don't think two people could have been happier till this terrible disease came.* I can't fight any longer. *I know that I am spoiling your life, that without me you could work.* And you will I know. You see I can't even write this properly. I can't read. What I want to say is I owe all the happiness of my life to you. You have been entirely patient with me and incredibly good. I want to say that—everybody knows it. If anybody could have saved me it would have been you. Everything has gone from me but the certainty of your goodness. I can't go on spoiling your life any longer. I don't think two people could have been happier than we have been. V.[13]

Dearest, I want to tell you that you have given me compete happiness. No one could have done more than you have. Please believe that. But I know that I shall never get over this: and I am wasting your life.... You can work, and you will be much better without me.... All I wish to say is that until this disease came on me we were perfectly happy. It was all due to you. No one could have been so good as you have been from the very first day till now. Everyone knows that. V.[14]

Dearest, I feel that I have gone too far this time to come back again. I am certain now that I am going mad again.... I am always hearing voices, and I know I shan't get over it now. I shan't recover this time.... All I want to say is that Leonard has been astonishingly good, every day, always.... We have been perfectly happy until the last few weeks, when this horror began.... *I feel he has so much to do that he will go on, better without me, and you will help him.* Virginia."[15]

Virginia's prediction about Leonard's future without her proved to be correct. He lived happily for another twenty-eight years.

Virginia's protestations of her happiness with Leonard ring hollow. They are inconsistent with her "psychotic symptoms" and with what we know about their life together. Several commentators have noticed this. Roger Poole writes: "It seems clear that Virginia regarded Leonard...[as] someone she hardly knew and who hardly knew her."[16] Alma Bond observes: "Virginia treated him [Leonard] as if his whole raison d'être was to perform as her adjunct."[17]

4

For twenty-nine years, Leonard Woolf watched his wife—like an anxious mother watches her sickly infant—ever on the alert for signs that she might kill herself. When he detected such a danger, he did what he thought was needed and enlisted professional help to prevent her from committing suicide. In March 1941, he stopped doing so. The steps he took were tokens, just enough to make him feel comfortable about not blaming himself, and assuring that he would not being blamed by others, for her death.

We have two rather different accounts of the last weeks of Virginia's life—one from Leonard, another from Bell. The last volume of

Leonard's autobiography was published in 1969, three years before Bell's biography of Virginia.

Leonard wrote: "There is a note in my diary on March 18 that she was not well and in the next week I became more and more alarmed. I am not sure whether early in that week she did not unsuccessfully try to commit suicide." He then describes Virginia coming home "soaking wet." He continued: "On Friday, March 21, Octavia came to tea and I told her that I thought Virginia on the verge of danger. On Monday, March 24, she was slightly better, but two days later I knew that the situation was very dangerous...she was terrified of madness. One knew that at any moment she might kill herself."[18] Leonard wrote as if he were observing the clinical course of severe malaria, the fever waxing and waning, with death lurking around the corner. But Virginia was not ill. She was tired of living, contemplating her own, self-inflicted death, as she had done many times before.

It was too late to stop. The show had to go on. "The only chance for her was to *give in and admit that she was ill, but this she would not do.*"[19] Leonard and Virginia were being impaled on their mendacious vocabulary. Months before, Virginia had told Octavia that she was afraid of "going mad." Throughout her life, Virginia accepted that going mad was a medical problem. What, then, did Leonard mean when he wrote that Virginia had to "give in and admit that she was ill"? She had frequently admitted that. She admitted it so completely that she concluded, as her doctors did also, that she was "incurable." The problem was not that she denied her "illness," as Leonard put it, and as psychiatrists love to put it. The problem was that she was a coward who preferred to frame her problematic life situation in terms of mental illness instead of framing it as the problem of what to do with the rest of her life.

The medicalization of Virginia's existential predicaments continued to the bitter end and beyond the grave. Leonard provides this account of the last weeks: "Octavia has been coming to see us about once a week, bringing cream and milk. *These visits were, so far as Virginia was concerned, just friendly visits, but I had told Octavia how serious I thought Virginia's condition was becoming and from our point of view, the visits were partly medical.*"[20] Leonard was shifting responsibility for Virginia's "medical care" to Octavia, whose double role as friend and denominated mad-doctor made her a perfect dupe. If Leonard thought Virginia to be on the verge of suicide, he could have insisted on taking her to Head in London or could have asked Octavia to commit her. He did neither.

At this point, Leonard acknowledged that his forcing Virginia to see Head in 1913 might have been a big mistake: "The memory of 1913 when the attempted suicide was the immediate result of the interview with Dr. Head haunted me."[21] It was too late. The die had been cast years ago. The time had passed for thinking clearly about whether psychiatry was the problem or the solution.

Using his newfound reconstruction of the tragedy of 1913, Leonard rationalized that recourse to psychiatry was now the source of danger: "We felt *it was not safe to do anything more at the moment. And it was the moment at which the risk had to be taken, for if one did not force the issue*—which would have meant perpetual surveillance of trained nurses—one would have made it impossible and intolerable to her if one attempted the same kind of perpetual surveillance by oneself. The decision was wrong, and led to the disaster."[22] Was the decision wrong? Was the result a disaster or a denouement desired by all, except perhaps Octavia, who was both naive and deep over her head in a long-standing marital-psychiatric drama?

Bell's account of Virginia's last days is briefer than Leonard's. His medicalization of the final decision-making is even more naive. To the bitter end, Bell wrote as if he believed that Virginia would have lived to a happy old age if only she had "admitted" that she was "mentally ill": "It was a symptom of Virginia's madness that she *could not admit* that she was mentally ill."[23] Inquisitors treated women accused of witchcraft with more dignity than Bell accorded Virginia. They would say that the witch *would not admit* that she was a witch. For someone allegedly so bereft of agency as Virginia, she did a very good job of killing herself.

The Woolf marriage—the drama of "me mad, you nurse"—had unwound. Scottish psychiatrist and psychobiographer I. Malcolm Ingram concludes:

> From these accounts an accurate diagnosis of her final illness can be made. From the suicide note alone, most psychiatrists would make a confident diagnosis of severe depression. She says that she is not only depressed, but going "mad" again; she is beginning to hear voices. She can't concentrate, can't read or write. She shows self-blame, believing that she is spoiling her husband's life.[24]

I believe that Virginia Woolf killed herself not because she was mad, but because she wanted to end her life. The way she killed herself is consistent with the view that she was a relentless self-dramatizer. Mad geniuses are supposed to commit suicide. Virginia's dramatic suicide affirmed and validated her genius (as well as her madness).

Virginia led a largely joyless life, her existence a burden rather than a challenge. She wanted to be famous. I surmise that she killed herself, and killed herself as she did, to enhance her fame. In adopting this tactic, she became a role model for mad-genius female writers and poets, such as Sylvia Plath and Anne Sexton, whose fame, like Virginia's, lies at least partly in their suicides.

In March 1941, in the middle of the war, Virginia was a lonely, aging woman. She neither loved nor liked Leonard. Vanessa had a busy life of her own. Virginia had never been close to Adrian or Karin. She had no children or grandchildren. No one needed her. She feared for her future and escaped it.[25]

What was Virginia Woolf afraid of? An empty, lonely, childless old age with a man whom she disliked? Literary impotence? Boredom? As usual, she said she feared going mad, her cop-out when faced with existential dilemmas. I don't know the answer. But I am confident she did not kill herself *because* she was "mad."

5

Before concluding this chapter, I think it might be worthwhile to take a brief critical look at why both mental health experts and intelligent laypersons remain squeamish about suicide and treat it as if it were a symptom of mental illness. I have examined this subject in detail elsewhere[26] and a few observations must suffice here.

What could be more "natural" than life and death? Why, then, do we speak of "unnatural death," why does the law recognize a category of *human* deaths as "unnatural," and why is suicide, along with homicide, considered "unnatural"? Clearly, we do not mean that there is anything literally unnatural about certain kinds of deaths; what we do mean is that we condemn the cause or mode by which death was brought about, and want to penalize, or at least criticize, the person who "caused" it, the "self-murderer." We blacken his name with a psychiatric label, or with an explicit moral condemnation, or both. The persistence of the term "unnatural"—to deligitimize, stigmatize, and prohibit certain kinds of deaths and sexual acts—reveals its roots in the monotheistic religions. Acts ostensibly legitimized by God are "natural," those not legitimized, "unnatural."[27] For example, in his *Summa Theologica*, Saint Thomas Aquinas (1225?-1274), asks, "Whether the unnatural vice is a species of lust?" and answers: "It would seem that the unnatural vice is not a species of lust…lust regards acts directed to human generation,…whereas the unnatural vice concerns acts from which generation cannot follow. Therefore the unnatural vice is not a species of lust."[28]

For centuries, Church and State severely condemned and harshly punished a vast range of non-procreative sexual acts as unnatural. A Christian website explains:

> Natural sexual activity are those acts between an adult male…and a female who has reached an age of sufficient maturity to responsibly bear children as God wills (husband and his wife).… All focused ejaculations of a human male must be deposited within the vagina of a mature human female. The activity may not have been intentionally rendered infertile either by the male or the female. A woman may only receive sperm from a human male in the approved natural manner. All other two party…sexual activity wherein one or both participants are human is condemned as unnatural.[29]

During the nineteenth century—in the Judeo-Christian West, but not in the Muslim East—most sexual acts hitherto classified as unnatural metamorphosed into mental illnesses (or their manifestations), justifying punishment in the disguise of psychiatric "intervention," "help," or "treatment."[30] Suicide—a grave sin in all three monotheistic religions—underwent a similar transformation, from wicked and unnatural, to sick or pathological.

Jurists, lawyers, and forensic pathologists still refer to some deaths as "unnatural." A group of forensic pathologists explain: "If the manner of death is unnatural, a medical examiner, coroner, or justice of the peace should certify the cause of death." When is the manner of death considered unnatural? Consistent with the pharmacratic ideology of our age, virtually all deaths that occur "without medical attendance" are regarded as suspicious and unexplained, hence potentially "unnatural." In this usage, the term is used prescriptively, not descriptively: It means that the death is reportable to the Medical Examiner; it does not mean that the death is not natural. Homicide and suicide (itself a species of homicide) are paradigmatic examples of "unnatural" (reportable) deaths.[31] It is worth noting that the requirement to report such deaths is not unreasonable.

Murder may be concealed as suicide, a theme that is a staple of murder mysteries.

Johann Wolfgang von Goethe (1749-1832) wisely observed, "Every suicide is an event that is a part of human nature. However much may have been said and done about it in the past, every person must confront it for himself anew, and every age must come to its own terms with it."[32] When Goethe was born, suicide was a moral-religious issue. By the time he died, it was on its way to becoming a medical-psychiatric problem, a symptom of madness.

Leslie Stephen struggled in print with the problem of the morality and legality of suicide. Virginia Woolf struggled with it in life. We are too cowardly and squeamish to even acknowledge that suicide is "an event that is a part of human nature" and look to psychiatrists to shield us from so "unnatural" an event.

7

"He's got a finger in my mind"

1

The fear of being invaded, penetrated, defiled—violated in body, mind, or spirit—played a crucial role at every juncture in Virginia's life, most notably in childhood and at the end of her life. It is the most constant and most characteristic feature of her personality and is consistent with her attitude toward psychoanalysis.

There is danger, in trying to understand Virginia Woolf, of overestimating the effects of childhood sexual violation on her. I believe that *every child is violated*, one way or another. It is the fate of being a child.

Dependent economically and physically on adults, the child is at the mercy of grown-ups and older children. Intrusion into his mind and body, in ways that the child may experience as a violation of his self, is intrinsic to childhood. Examples of such (actual or potential) violations include countless experiences—familial, educational, religious, and medical—*to which the child is compelled to submit*. In this wider but nonetheless relevant sense, every child is the victim of "abuse." As adults, it is our duty to strive to overcome and cope with the deleterious effects of our particular victimization. It is a grave mistake, in my view, to divide people into two groups: one comprising individuals who are the victims of childhood (sexual) "abuse," another comprising individuals free of such victimization.

I say this not to belittle the significance of Virginia's traumatic childhood sexual experiences, nor the significance of different degrees and kinds of violations and victimizations in general. I say it to emphasize that the impact of the violation depends also on the child's age, biological constitution, family situation, subsequent experiences, and perhaps most importantly, on how she (or he) constructs the meaning of the violation and on how she wants to use or not use the memory of the violation in living her life.

Virginia and her biographers agree that her half-brothers, George and Gerald Duckworth, displayed inappropriate sexual interest in both Vanessa and Virginia. In *A Sketch of the Past*, written only two years before she killed herself, Virginia reminisced: "I can remember the feel of his [Gerald's] hands going under my clothes; going firmly and steadily lower and lower, I remember how I hoped that he would stop; how I stiffened and wriggled as his hand approached my private parts. But he did not stop."[1]

Vanessa was probably subjected to similar experiences. What effect they had on her we do not know. She never complained about them. For Virginia, however, George Duckworth's sexual interest in her body came to symbolize having to submit to a male, being humiliated and violated. She continued to interpret a long series of events and experiences in this light—for example, Vanessa's teasing and tormenting her, when they were children; pious relatives' haranguing her about religion, when she was an adolescent; men's expecting to have sexual relations with her, when she became an adult and after she married; physicians', especially psychiatrists', ordering her about, during much of her life; and, finally, the threat of Nazi invasion of England, when she killed herself.

Still, after all is said and done, Virginia was, as we all are, responsible for how she framed her childhood and lived her life. On January 12, 1941, barely two months before she killed herself, she still dwelled on her having been molested: "I still shiver with shame at the memory of my half-brother standing me on a ledge, aged about 6 or so, exploring my private parts."[2] Virginia was then fifty-nine years old. England was being bombarded by the *Luftwaffe* and she feared that the country was about to be invaded by the Nazis. If Virginia still shivered at *this* thought, at *this* time, it was because she treasured it as a memory justifying the lifestyle she had chosen for herself, and with the consequences of which she was now stuck.

2

Virginia Woolf's deeply ingrained habit of protecting her body and soul from the Other permeated every aspect of her life, especially her supposedly most intimate relationships. Victoria Glendinning, in her excellent, definitive biography of Victoria (Vita)

Sackville-West—Virginia's supposed lesbian lover—cites Vita as chiding her friend: "I believe you look upon everything, human relationships included…'as copy' [i.e. material for a next book]…. Do you ever mean what you say, or say what you mean? or do you just enjoy baffling people who try to creep a little nearer?"[3]

Vita was ten years younger than Virginia but was a far more fully developed person. She was successfully married to Harold Nicolson, a prominent diplomat (and a homosexual, like herself), the mother of two sons, an award-winning poet and author, and the proprietor of Knole House in Kent, one of the most famous country homes and gardens in England. Vita, who probably knew Virginia better than anyone else, believed that "Virginia's experience of close physical contact was limited. She had no sexual life with Leonard. She was clever, critical, ironic, mischievous even—yet ever so nervous, fantastical, childlike, that even a kiss or a caressing hand might seem sensational to her. 'I was always sexually cowardly,' she would write."[4]

Did Virginia have a lesbian relationship with Vita, as many biographers believe? Not according to Vita: "Imagine my horror when he [Clive Bell] suddenly said 'I wonder if I dare ask Vita a very indiscreet question?' and I, being innocent and off my guard, said yes he might, and he came out with 'Have you ever gone to bed with Virginia?' but I think my 'NEVER!' convinced him and everybody else of its truth."[5] It did not. Perhaps in an effort to humanize and normalize Virginia, most writers assert or imply that Virginia succumbed to Vita's sexual overtures. It seems unlikely.

3

Dwelling on the traumatic effects of sexual abuse on children, especially female children, has been fashionable since Freud's days and is now *de rigeur* in feminist and psychiatric literature. Although much has been made of Virginia's violation by George Duckworth, she had also been subjected to a very different kind of violation that—according to her own account and in my opinion—imbued her with far more intense animus against the aggressors than she had felt against her molesting half-brother.

Since this violation involves religion, not sex, Virginia's biographers have, unsurprisingly, virtually ignored it. The very possibility of such a thing as the *religious abuse of a child* is *interdit* in polite company, especially in the faith-intoxicated atmosphere of the United States today. However, I believe we should consider the possibility that Virginia suffered more from religious abuse than she did from sexual abuse.

Sir Leslie Stephen was not only an eminent Victorian, he was also an eminent atheist. His children were not baptized and were raised as atheists, which set them apart from the norm. They were religious deviants, subject to religious harassment. Again, there is no evidence that Vanessa was so traumatized. But Virginia was. In a letter to Ethel Smyth, dated May 18, 1931, she describes the religious abuse to which she has been subjected, the memory of which evidently was never far from her mind:

> I never pass through Hyde Park without cursing separately every God inventor there. This partly because, unbaptized as we were, our religious friends, some cousins in particular, the daughters of Fitzjames, rasped and agonized us as children by perpetual attempts at conversion. As they were ugly women, who sweated, *I conceived a greater hatred for them than ever for anyone.* And even now, when no one tries, I still draw in and shiver at the suspicion— *he's got a finger in my mind.*[6]

There is an intensity of hatred and fear in these words that far surpasses anything that Virginia said to anyone (as far as we know) about George Duckworth.

No one was going to have a finger in Virginia Woolf's mind, ever! Nor was anyone ever going to introduce anything into any part of her body that she herself did not want introduced. It seems simple— and she made it clear enough in *Mrs. Dalloway*—but no one around Virginia wanted to hear it. And Virginia made no effort to explain herself. Doing so would have implied a desire to come to terms with her past traumatic experiences, something she did not want to do.

In *Mrs. Dalloway*, Virginia Woolf makes her key traumatic experience explicit: Sir William Bradshaw was "a great doctor yet obscurely evil...extremely polite to women, but capable of some indescribable outrage—*forcing your soul, that was it.*"[7] The same image recurs in her description of psychoanalysis, where she describes seeing "a woman in the last agony of despair," and her psychoanalyst brother as a "vulture."[8] Virginia "saw" no such thing. She saw a sad woman, not a woman in her last agony. And she saw her brother, not a vulture.

Sigmund Freud wanted to penetrate the soul to uncover its secrets. Virginia Woolf wanted to protect the soul and its secrets from prying eyes. She comprehended and conveyed to us, as few others have, the perils of being understood, of having what we now call "good human relationships." Writers of popular songs have long rhapsodized over lovers who never separate. Virginia wrote to Lytton Strachey, probably the only man she ever truly loved, other than her father: "Find me a house where no one can ever come."[9] She was then in the thirteenth year of her marriage to Leonard Woolf, who had so protectively, yet violently, shared her house—though not "that snowfield of the [her] mind, where man has not trodden."[10]

In the little gem of a book, *On Being Ill*, Virginia Woolf comes close to revealing her deepest longings and hence her true self:

> We do not know our own souls, let alone the souls of others. Human beings do not go hand in hand the whole stretch of the way. There is a virgin forest in each; a snow field where even the birds' feet is unknown. Here we go alone, and like it better so. Always to have sympathy, always to be accompanied, always to be understood would be intolerable. But in health the genial pretense must be kept up and the effort renewed—to communicate, to civilize, to share, to cultivate the desert, educate the native, to work together by day and by night to sport. In illness this make-believe ceases…we cease to be soldiers in the army of the upright; we become deserters.[11]

Appendix I

Virginia Woolf, Mad Genius

1

My interpretation of Virginia Woolf's life and work as expressions of her character, and of her character as the "product" of her free will, is intended, in part, as a corrective against the prevailing, ostensibly scientific view that attributes both her "madness" and her "genius" to biological-genetic causes.[1] In this Appendix, I offer examples of, and excerpts from, the works of authors who endorse the latter view.

The belief that there are subtle but significant connections between illness and greatness—the former enhancing or causing the latter—goes back to antiquity. Abraham J. Heschel (1907-1972), a distinguished professor at the Jewish Theological Seminary of America, notes: "The Greek word for prophecy (*mantike*), and the word for madness (*manike*) were really the same, and the letter *t* is only an insertion."[2] Aristotle thought the poet is *manikos*, afflicted with madness.

The first ailment known to be linked with genius was epilepsy, the "sacred disease" of the ancients. Since antiquity, believers in the mythology of illness-as-inspiration have supported their faith by producing rosters of famous people afflicted with their favorite creativity-genic disease, from epilepsy to tuberculosis, syphilis, alcoholism, and, currently, manic-depression. The standard list of famous epileptics includes Alexander the Great, Socrates, Julius Caesar, Saint Paul, Joan of Arc, Molière, Cardinal Richelieu, Napoleon Bonaparte, Edgar Allan Poe, Pope Pius IX, Vincent van Gogh, Gustave Flaubert, Fyodor Dostoyevsky, Charles Dickens, Alfred Nobel, Vladimir Ilyich Lenin, and Margaux Hemingway.[3]

The supposed linkage between epilepsy and greatness remained popular until the nineteenth century, when it was displaced by the supposed linkage between tuberculosis and genius. The standard list of famous persons with tuberculosis includes: Jane Austen, Honoré de Balzac, Frédéric Bartholdi, Frédéric Bastiat, Alexander Graham Bell, Simon Bolivar, Louis Braille, Elizabeth Barrett Browning, Emily Bronte, Charlotte Bronte, John Calvin, Albert Camus, Anders Celsius, Stephen Crane, Anton Checkov, Frederick Chopin, Ralph Waldo Emerson, Stephen Foster, Paul Gauguin, Johann Wolfgang von Goethe, Washington Irving, Samuel Johnson, Immanuel Kant, Franz Kafka, John Keats, René Théophile Hyacinthe Laennec, D.H. Lawrence, Vivien Leigh, Nelson Mandela, Thomas Mann, Katherine Mansfield, Somerset Maugham, Guy de Maupassant, Eugene O'Neill, George Orwell, Niccolo Paganini, Walker Percy, Alexander Pope, Edmond Rostand, Jean-Jacques Rousseau, John Ruskin, Friedrich Schiller, Erwin Schrödinger, Sir Walter Scott, Baruch Spinoza, Laurence Sterne, Robert Louis Stevenson, Henry David Thoreau, Desmond Tutu, and Lev Vygotsky.[4]

Today, the illness that "explains" both madness (bad habit, misbehavior, crime, suicide) and genius (exceptional achievement, great art) is mental illness, especially manic-depression (also called bipolar illness).

2

One of the best-known proponents of the view that Virginia Woolf was the victim of manic-depression and that manic-depression is a genetic and creativity-genic disease is Kay Redfield Jamison. Her popularity rests in large part on her dual role as mental health professional and mental patient: She is a psychologist, a professor of psychiatry at Johns Hopkins University medical school, and a "genius" authenticated by the MacArthur Foundation. In addition, Jamison is a self-declared mental patient: She claims to have been psychotically depressed and to have attempted suicide, and now claims to be "exuberant." A report in *U.S. News & World Report* characterizes Jamison as follows: "The dual perspective of expert and afflicted endow author, psychologist, and manic-depressive Kay Redfield Jamison, 55, with a sharp perspective on mood disorders and suicide."[5] In an interview with *Psychiatric Times*,

Jamison claimed that speaking about her illness has allowed her to speak her mind more freely on other topics as well. She quipped, "Everybody thinks

I'm crazy anyway...I am much more able to say what I really feel now." Writing about her illness brought Jamison's family closer together. She said they have begun talking about the prevalence of manic depression among themselves—a topic they had ignored before. She described her family tree as "very loaded—as they say in genetics."[6]

Jamison has no valid claim to expertise in medicine or genetics: She is neither a physician nor a geneticist. Her career as a manic-depressive, suicidal-exuberant mental patient does not provide her, popular opinion notwithstanding, with medical or genetic expertise. Since Jamison uses her own alleged "suicide attempts" as professional credential, we are entitled to conclude that, for an expert on suicide, she is not very good at it. The term "suicide" means killing oneself, not dramatizing oneself.

Physicians are human and suffer from all the diseases that afflict non-physicians. Medical authorities and the media do not regard a physician who happens to have, say, glaucoma as, ipso facto, an expert on the disease. The opposite is the case with respect to persons who suffer from mental diseases, especially "depression." If such an individual docilely submits to psychiatric diagnosis, praises the drug treatment that "controls his illness," and becomes an active promoter of the psychiatric ideology, mental health professionals and media pundits hail her or him as an expert, possessing special insight into the "disease" and its proper "treatment." Jane Pauley and William Styron, poster persons for the miracle cures of modern biological psychiatry, are examples. At the same time, ordinary men and women who denounce forced psychiatric drugging and organize protest groups against psychiatric deprivations of liberty are dismissed as "sickos" lacking insight into their illnesses.

Jamison is certain that Virginia Woolf and countless other artists have suffered from manic-depression and that manic-depression is a genetically determined brain disease that "causes" suicide. With sovereign disregard for evidence, Jamison's confidence in her post-mortem diagnoses and in the neurological basis of the condition she calls "manic-depression" is not tempered by Virginia Woolf's long medical history. Virginia had been examined by several prominent English neurologists, among them Sir Henry Head, a giant in the field. *None found her to be suffering from a neurological illness.*

Virginia's family, husband, friends, and biographers looked at her and saw an irritable, brittle, chronically sad woman, perpetually on the verge of a "breakdown" and suicide. James King, the author of a monumental (699-page) biography of Virginia Woolf, writes: "Her entire life was dominated by depression and sadness..."[7] Jamison looks at her and beholds a joyous and fearless adventurer, a literary Joan of Arc, blessed with "exuberance": "With the breath of voices in her sails, Virginia Woolf lived her life as a journey from one great individual moment to the next."[8] Mental patients *hallucinate*. Virginia Woolf had *"the breath of voices in her sails."*

Jamison is persuaded that manic-depression is a brain disease that "enhances creativity," and she is eager to persuade others: "[O]ne way of looking at it [manic-depression] is that *there is something that is added*. Say you're creative.... Is something added to that that makes it different because you have a mood disorder? *I think absolutely, unequivocally yes.*"[9] Jamison cites Virginia Woolf in support: "[Virginia] believed unequivocally in the importance of melancholia and madness to her imaginative powers."[10] As we have seen, Virginia Woolf believed that she was ill or not ill as suited her purpose.

Lest the reader be left with the impression that the "effective treatment" of manic-depression diminishes creativity, Jamison is ready with the antidote, the "studies" made to order: "There have been two studies that have asked artists and writers, 'Are you as productive on lithium as you were before, or not as productive, or more productive?' Three quarters of artists and writers say they are as productive or more productive."[11] Not long ago, the term "study" referred to scholarly investigation committed to truth-telling; today, it is likely to refer to professionally authenticated lies and propaganda.

Jamison dwells lovingly on the suicides of the artists whose lives and deaths she uses to spin her fantasies about the creativity-genic effects of bipolar illness. Although she claims to be pleased with having this affliction, she hastens to reassure the reader that she is not recommending the disease to her family: "But do you want your child to have it?... Absolutely no.... *Do I want my nephews and niece to have to go through this?* Absolutely no.... [O]ne out of four or five untreated manic-depressive individuals actually does commit suicide."[12]

Jamison regards mental illness as a "fatal disease," emphasizes the importance of suicide prevention, and identifies herself as a mental patient. She asserts that the distinction between voluntary and involuntary psychiatric relations is "misleading and arbitrary,"[13] and characterizes herself as someone who may, at any moment, re-lapse into psychosis and become legally incompetent: "I drew up a clear arrangement with my psychiatrist and family that if I again become severely depressed they have the authority to approve, against my will if necessary, both electroconvulsive therapy, or ECT, an excellent treatment for certain types of severe depression, and hospitalization."[14] Although Jamison attributes her recovery from manic-depression to lithium, here she does not even mention the drug.

In March 2003, Jamison addressed "more than 500 residency training directors at the annual meeting of the American Association of Directors of Psychiatric Residency Training." Based on her own personal experiences as a bipolar patient on lithium, she rec-ommended "Rules for the Gracious Acceptance of Lithium Into Your Life," including the following: "Clear out the medicine cabinet before guests come for dinner or new lovers stay the night. Remember to put the lithium back in the cabinet the next day. Don't be too embarrassed by your lack of coordination.... Try not to let the fact that you can't read without effort annoy you. Be philosophical. Even if you could read, you couldn't remember most of it anyway."[15]

Jamison's views on the supposed connections between manic-depression and creativity are devoid of evidence. "There are some people," she tells us, "who *feel* [sic] that Mozart had manic de-pression. And Beethoven...it certainly *seems* to be the case, from 20, 25 studies, that there's a much higher rate of depression and manic-depression in highly creative artists, writers and compos-ers."[16] How people *feel* about other persons or how other persons *seem* to them are not medical methods for determining *what ill-ness, if any, these (medically unexamined individuals) have.* Jamison cites no statistics about the rate of depression in "uncre-ative people," for the simple reason that most psychiatrists are not interested in them.

Most people view the diagnostic label of manic-depression as a stigma. Jamison treats it as an honorific and uses it to bolster her credentials and credibility as an expert on mental illness and psy-chiatric coercion. Although she is neither an artist nor a scientist, she is widely regarded as an expert on the scientific (psychiatric) understanding of art. Science writer Jo-Ann C. Gutin is not taken in. In a skeptical essay titled, "The Science of Creativity," she writes:

Even the most ardent advocates of the connection concede that most creativity has nothing to do with mental illness and that most of the mentally ill, bipolar or otherwise, are no more creative than the rest of us.... Johns Hopkins University psychologist Kay Redfield Jamison, whose many books and articles on the subject have made her the de facto point person for the art-and-madness link, has compiled a roll call of the artists in this unhappy club that reads like the A-list for the cocktail party of the millennium. Among them are poets William Blake, John Keats, Percy Bysshe Shelley, Edgar Allan Poe, Emily Dickinson, and Anne Sexton; novelists Emile Zola, Mary Shelley, Leo Tolstoy, Maxim Gorky, and Robert Louis Stevenson; playwright Eugene O'Neill; visual artists Michelangelo, Theodore Gericault, Edvard Munch, Paul Gaughin, Vincent van Gogh, Mark Rothko, and Georgia O'Keeffe; and musicians from Handel to Charlie Parker. She includes, in fact, practically every famously tormented artist in the canon...when Kay Jamison talks about the effects of bipolar disease, she sounds downright mystical.[17]

However, the media love Jamison's dramatic self-representations, ranging from expert on depression and suicide, to expert on exuberance and the celebration of life. Interviewed in the *Washington Post* about her new book, *Exuberance*, she explains: "Exuberance binds us to life, and to the future..."[18] False. What binds us to life is the inertia of living, the "hard-wired" instinct to avert dying, work, and our ties to people we love and to whom we have obligations. But never mind. Jamison is not talking about what binds us to life. She is talking about her favorite subject, herself.

"So you are exuberant?" the reporter asks. Jamison replies: "Oh, yeah, yeah, yeah! I've always seen life as fantastic. I couldn't wait to get up in the morning, didn't want to go to sleep at night, had a lot of things I wanted to do.... All my life I've been very exuberant by temperament." Having renamed the manic part of *her* manic-depression "exuberance," Jamison thinks she has made a discovery. She explains: "That's a terribly important aspect of exuberance. Many do have both sides. Like Virginia Woolf—I get so sick of writers and film makers painting her as a doomed character. She was not a gloomy, doomy person. *She had a bad disease*, but for the most part she was vivacious, filled with laughter, had a wicked wit."[19]

3

Jamison is a major player in psychiatry's anti-suicide propaganda campaign. She uses the term "suicide prevention" as if the psychiatric coercions to which she refers would in fact be effective measures for preventing suicide. The evidence indicates the opposite: Psychiatric suicide prevention tends to inflame the subject's desire to kill himself; suicide hotlines increase the incidence of suicide. [20] Nevertheless, Jamison mendaciously declares, "The decision to admit a suicidal patient to a psychiatric hospital is often straightforward and reassuring to all concerned."[21] It is not reassuring to the imprisoned victim who often responds to it by killing himself. My source for the following statistic is Jamison's own text, coauthored with Goodwin: "[One psychiatrist] found that 7 percent of the patients in their sample had committed suicide *while in a psychiatric hospital*. [Another] reported an even higher rate: 27 percent of manic-depressive patients killed themselves *while under hospital care*."[22] Six pages later, the authors shamelessly declare, "Treatment of manic-depressive illness remains one of the true successes of modern medicine."[23]

In her defense of psychiatry, Jamison does not hesitate to assert brazen falsehoods. In *Touched With Fire*, she declares, "Artists and writers, like everyone else, ultimately decide for themselves whether or not, and how, to be treated."[24] She knows this is not true. The index to her book lists six references to the French writer, Antonin Artaud (1896-1948), but she does not mention his famous *cri de coeur:* "I myself spent nine years in an insane asylum and I never had the obsession of suicide, but I know that each conversation with a psychiatrist, every morning at the time of his visit, made me want to hang myself, realizing that I would not be able to slit his throat."[25]

Analyzing the case of Ernest Hemingway (1899-1961), Jamison presents a genealogical table of four generations, comprising thirteen individuals, three of whom she claims suffered from manic-depression, and four of whom died by suicide.[26] She says nothing about Hemingway the person or why he decided to kill himself. If we want to understand why Hemingway killed himself and why he did so when he did, we must know who he was and the circumstances that led to his suicide. As the fragility of glass doesn't explain why a glass vase breaks, so genes and manic-depression cannot explain why a person kills himself.

From his teens, Hemingway chose to lead a juvenile-macho life of dramatic action and of excitement engendered by danger. Before the United States entered World War I, he saw action in Europe as a volunteer in an ambulance corps. He covered the Spanish Civil War and World War II as a reporter. He married four times. He "was widely quoted as saying, 'My writing is nothing. My boxing is everything.'"[27] Self-discipline, self-reflection, temperance, and kindness were not in Hemingway's nature. "My father," he said, "was a coward. He shot himself without necessity."[28] How does such an unfeeling, unreflective, unkind person age? Not well.

In his definitive biography of his friend, A. E. Hotchner's relates many of the *human reasons* for Hemingway's suicide—as against the *supposed genetic-medical determinants of his alleged manic-depression that caused his suicide.* In December 1960, Hemingway's fourth wife, journalist Mary Welsh, became seriously concerned that he was about to kill himself. She prevailed on him to admit himself to a famous medical center. Once admitted, he was incarcerated in the psychiatric unit. Hotchner, a close friend of Hemingway's, writes: "Ernest was not permitted to receive or make phone calls.... During the month of December [1960], Ernest was given eleven treatments with electric shock."[29]

Hotchner visited Hemingway, who told him: "Well, what is the sense of ruining my head and erasing my memory, which is my capital, and putting me out of business? It was a brilliant cure but we lost the patient. It's a bum turn, Hotch, terrible."[30]

Hemingway was released and returned to Idaho with Mary. Three months later, Mary was more alarmed than ever. Refusing further psychiatric interference in his life, Hemingway was overpowered, drugged, and put on a private plane headed back to the clinic. En route, he attempted to jump from the plane. Back at the clinic, he was incarcerated and given more ECT against his will. Mary told Hotchner: "What alarms me, though, is his talk about returning home. One thing I am sure of is that a repetition of the last three months would destroy me in one way or another."[31] This brief remark exposes the true reason for Hemingway's involuntary mental hospitalization and treatment: because his wife could not stand being in the same house with him. A wife's leaving such a "sick husband" is unseemly. What is seemly is having him psychiatrically tortured and destroyed, in the name of his health. Manic-depression is the medical-therapeutic rationalization and justification for assault and battery against the "patient."

Hotchner continues: "During the month of May [1961], Ernest received a number of electrical treatments.... She [Mary] reported that Ernest was even more infuriated with these treatments than the previous ones, registering even bitterer complaints about how his memory was wrecked and how he was ruined as a writer and putting the blame for all this on the [medical center] doctors."[32]

Hotchner tells the story and refrains from interpretation: "Mary asked, 'How can we make him see the extent of his problem...?' "[33] It was, of course, Mary who had a problem. Ernest Hemingway had a solution. Hotchner asked him: "'Papa, why do you want to kill yourself?' He hesitated only a moment; then he spoke in his old, deliberate way: 'Hotch, if I can't exist on my own terms, then existence is impossible.... What does a man care about? Staying healthy. Working good. Eating and drinking with his friends. Enjoying himself in bed. I haven't any of them. Do you understand, goddamn it? None of them.'"[34] Hotchner adds: "He was a man of prowess, and he could not live without it: writing prowess, physical prowess, sexual prowess, drinking and eating prowess."[35] Hemingway is discharged, returns to his home in Idaho, and shoots himself in the head with one of his guns.

4

The views of other psychiatrically (mis)informed writers more or less rehash the arguments advanced by Jamison. Thomas C. Caramagno—a professor of English and author of *The Flight of the Mind: Virginia Woolf's Art and ManicDepressive Illness*—regards himself as a disciple of Jamison's. He states: "In this interdisciplinary study of Virginia Woolf, I reexamine her madness and her fiction in the light of recent discoveries about the biological basis of manic-depressive illness—findings allied with drug therapies that today help nearly one million American manic-depressives to live happier, more productive lives."[36] Caramagno is a naively unabashed psychiatric propagandist.[37] The following passage is typical:

> Psychobiographers ignore psychobiology, in part because they are afraid of having to undertake a whole new program of self-education—reading dense biological texts.... In the 1960's, psychologists, pharmacologists, and psychiatrists joined forces in the expanding field of psychopharmacology, and by 1969 enough genetic and pharmacological evidence had been accumulated to persuade the American Psychiatric Association to recommend lithium to the Food and Drug Administration for treatment of manic-depressive illness. Today over 700,000 manic-depressive Americans take lithium. Further evidence came in 1987 when the first gene implicated in the transmission of the illness was identified, a discovery predicted by biochemical theory.... *We literary scholars can no longer afford to remain comfortably ignorant of the mechanisms of the brain...*[38]

Equipped with his newfound knowledge of "psychobiology," Caramagno has his own idiosyncratic interpretation of the Woolf marriage: "Leonard and Virginia's relationship was above all comradely: deeply affectionate and indivisibly united, they depended on each other."[39] Unfortunately, it is simply not true that Leonard depended on Virginia. After she died, he lived happily for another twenty-eight years, precisely as Virginia predicted in her suicide note. It is also not true that the relationship between Virginia and Leonard was comradely. Caramagno himself describes the relationship as similar to that between a protective mother and her sickly child:

> Leonard never failed in vigilance and never fussed; neither did he hide his brief anxiety that Virginia might drink a glass too much wine or commit some other mild excess; he would say quite simply, "Virginia, that's enough," and that was the end of it. Or, when he noticed by the hands of his enormous watch that it was 11:00 in the evening, no matter how much she was enjoying herself, he would say, "Virginia, we must go home," and after a few extra minutes stolen from beneath his nose, she would rise and...follow him and Pinka to the door.... To some readers, Leonard's behavior looks petty and tyrannical, but since alcohol, fatigue, and changes in sleep patterns do affect a manic-depressive's vulnerability to breakdowns.... It is unfortunate that *in this particular case it is the woman depending on the man (who acts as the restraining authority), for that inflames the readers who are justifiably moved by Virginia's eloquent appeals for women's liberation.*[40]

Caramagno concludes: "This intersection between literary theory and scientific inquiries may eventually lead us to a new model of the human psyche, one that integrates the valuable insights of psychoanalysis and neuroscience, mind and brain, Freud and Woolf."[41] The promise of "a new model of the human psyche, one that integrates the valuable insights of psychoanalysis and neuroscience, mind and brain" sounds inspiring, uplifting, altogether wonderful. But what does it mean? What would it be good for?

The myth of the creativity-genic nature of manic-depression is now so powerful that it attracts a steady flow of quacks eager to stake a claim in it. Alice Weaver Flaherty, author of *The Midnight Disease: The Drive to Write, Writer's Block, and the Creative Brain*, is a Harvard neurologist. Her other credentials for addressing the neuropathology of "writing" include two periods of psychiatric incarceration and the claim that she herself suffers from the disease she has invented. The dust jacket of *The Midnight Disease* states: "What underlies the human ability, desire, and even compulsion to write? Alice Flaherty first explores the brain state called hypergraphia—the overwhelming desire to write—and the science behind its antithesis, writer's block."[42]

These two sentences condense and convey the book's fatal defects: The term "hypergraphia" is listed in neither *Webster's Unabridged International Dictionary* nor the *Oxford English Dictionary*. Like most Greco-Latin psychiatric diagnostic terms, hypergraphia implies that a certain behavior or behavior pattern is a pathological phenomenon, a medical (mental) disease.[43] Flaherty asserts, without evidence, that "it" is a "brain state," characterized by an "overwhelming desire to write." Desires are subjective experiences. They are neither brain states nor diseases. If they were, then intense desires for chocolates, sex, money, travel, and every other "intense" human desire would be diseases. For thousands of years, moralists and religious leaders viewed desires as corrupting passions that individuals as moral agents must learn to control, perhaps even extinguish.

If hypergraphia is "the overwhelming desire to write," then its opposite is the lack of desire to write, not writer's block. If the disease is called "hypergraphia," then its opposite ought to be called "hypographia," not "writer's block." Furthermore, a writer with writer's block does not experience hypographia, that is, a diminished desire to write. On the contrary, he experiences an especially intense *desire* to write, but is *unable to write*. He resembles the man who has an intense desire to have sexual intercourse with a woman, but cannot get an erection. The level of ignorance—of Latin, logic, and the nuances of the English language—displayed in these few sentences does not inspire confidence in the author's medical competence.

Indeed, Flaherty parades ignorance as expertise. She writes: "As a doctor, I hope I do not simply see normal problems as illness; I want also to see that illness is often nearly normal. If we are all a little bit sick, it is not all that sick to be sick. Illness is even sometimes useful."[44] Flaherty conflates and confuses several distinct concepts and categories, such as disease as bodily lesion or biological condition, the sick role and its benefits ("secondary gain"), and normality as conformity and abnormality as deviance.

The terms "problem," "disease," and "normal" belong to different descriptive and logical categories. Assault is a problem—for the assaulted individual and his family. Malaria is a disease—and may or may not be a problem for the affected individual; in a group where everyone has malaria, members of the group may consider malaria normal, but for the pathologist it is still a disease.[45] Flaherty says, "I want also to see that illness is often nearly normal." If a person wants to see something badly, he'll see it. This is why people see statues of Mary, the mother of Jesus, shedding tears; why, until recently, psychiatrists saw homosexuality as an illness; and why Flaherty sees that "illness is nearly normal." She does exactly what she denies doing: She medicalizes human behavior and normalizes-romanticizes what psychiatrists call "psychotic behavior."

It gets worse: "Many readers, while granting that our minds are the products of our brains, believe that there are some aspects of our thoughts...that come from the outside." Flaherty does not tell us which "thoughts" or "aspects of thoughts" come from the outside and which do not; nor does she tells us where "from the outside"—or "inside"—they come from. What she does tell us is that she wants to obfuscate and obliterate the distinction between disease and health, ostensibly to understand them: "While doctors care about disease *because they want to cure* it, many neuroscientists care about disease *as a scalpel with which to dissect health.*"[46]

When I went to medical school, there were few diseases physicians could treat, much less cure. In those days, a great doctor was a great diagnostician. Yet, in those bygone days—before doctors could cure with antibiotics, steroids, statins, and beta blockers—doctors "cared" more about patients than they do now. Flaherty has a flair for making a point by resting it on a patent falsehood.

5

When Flaherty was first incarcerated in a madhouse, she was ignorant of the most elementary facts about psychiatry. She still is: "My husband and my psychiatrist, skeptical of my enlightenment and not persuaded by my notion that mental illness is sometimes preferable to sanity, eventually convinced me to go to a psychiatric hospital.... *I physically could not leave.* When I signed the standard voluntary admission papers that require a three-day review after a request for discharge, *I had no idea of the claustrophobia this provision would bring.* There was nothing wrong with the hospital."[47]

Even after being incarcerated, Flaherty still thinks that mental hospitals are bona fide hospitals: "Psychiatric hospitals are not terrible places to write—they bear certain similarities to writers' colonies like Yaddo, except that health insurance pays." She is oblivious of individual liberty and personal responsibility. Two hundred pages later, Flaherty is once again "hospitalized." This is her account of how she dealt with that encounter: "... [T]he admitting resident asked me a rote [sic] question about my self-image, and I described how my hands seemed alien, how they looked like leather claws, but how I knew this was a fancy;... He wrote 'psychotic' on the intake form and put me on a locked ward."[48] What did she expect he would write?

Undeterred by this evidence, the science writer for *U.S. News & World Report* believes Flaherty has actually discovered a new disease: "Clinically termed hypergraphia, the driving compulsion to write was shared by such geniuses as Fyodor Dostoevsky and Sylvia Plath.... Flaherty has written *The Midnight Disease* (Houghton Mifflin), in which she joins her scientific expertise with her experiences both as a writer and as a sufferer of mental illness, exploring the two extremes of the creative process: hypergraphia and its polar opposite, writer's block."[49]

Replying to the reporter's question, "Do you think that psychiatric treatment might stifle creativity?" Flaherty states: "I think it's important to talk about *the benefits of the mild versions of these disorders. But that's not to say that illness is good.... I present myself in the book as if I am all cured. But in fact, I am not all that cured. I am just better able to modulate. And my main fear is that I do get completely cured.*"[50]

In an interview in *Harvard Magazine*, Flaherty explains: "[W]riting, and not being able to write when you want to, come from interactions between and changes in specific areas of the brain. *The muse, in other words, is merely a matter of making the right brain connections.* The limbic system, a ringshaped cluster of cells deep in the brain, provides the emotional push.... Finally, the frontal lobe, behind your forehead, serves as a critical organizer and editor, penciling out bad phrases and ideas."[51] Again, metaphors masquerade as scientific explanations: muses are brain connections, editors are frontal lobes. Was lobotomy the mass murder of "editors"?

To diagnose a bodily disease, doctors examine the bodies of their patients and use objective measurements, called tests, of pathological bodily changes. Neuroscientists don't need tests: They can diagnose mental illness, creativity, and genius in long-dead poets and painters just by looking at their work. Moreover, their science is synonymous with therapy or "help." Flaherty declares: "Although creativity is transcendent, it is also, paradoxically, immanent—*something science can help.*"[52]

In physics, the term "science" refers to information about *how things are.* Scientists and science writers know that the fruits of real science may be useful for helping people or for harming them. In psychiatry, the term "neuroscience" refers to justifications for coercions that "can help." They cannot harm. Sounds familiar.

6

"When I was an adolescent my mother was mad.... Her particular madness manifested itself in what was *called* depression."[53] So begins *Women's Madness: Misogyny or Mental Illness?* by Jane M. Ussher, professor and head of the department of Women's Health Psychology at the University of Western Sydney in Australia. In addition to notes at the end of each chapter, there is a bibliography of twenty-three pages. Although the book appears to be a scholarly work, it is nothing of the sort. It is a mixture of catharsis, exhibitionism, psychiatric apologetics, and anti-male and anti-capitalist screed.

Ussher describes her mother as having been overwhelmed and depressed by domestic duties, suicidal, involuntarily hospitalized, and treated against her will with ECT and drugs. "Nearly twenty years later all this seems a distant memory.... She is happy, healthy, and independent, having escaped from many of the bonds that tied her."[54] Ussher herself has had a harder time overcoming her own problems. She writes: "I studied psychology: this would be where I would find the answers. Nine years of undergraduate, postgraduate research, and clinical psychology training equipped me with the academic armor with which to enter professional debates on the subject. But do I now have the answers? Unfortunately, I do not."[55] It does not seem to occur to Ussher that studying clinical psychology has *disabled* her not just from "having the answers" but also from knowing the questions.

Understandably, Ussher was eager to avoid suffering her mother's fate. Instead of becoming a mental patient, she became a mental heath professional. Naively, she declares: "This knowledge gives me power. I can now use my hard-earned skills to treat other women (and men) deemed mad.... I can intervene in their pain, as the psychiatrist treating my mad, sad mother did all those years ago."[56]

Ussher would have learned more about "madness" if instead of studying psychology, she had studied slavery. She would have learned, and perhaps learned from, Lincoln's famous *cri de coeur:* "As I would not be a slave, so I would not be a master. This expresses my idea of democracy." As it is, Ussher does not understand that having power over mental patients precludes helping them.

Ussher wanted to be an oppressor, and she got her wish. As a result, she is blind to personal liberty, individual responsibility, contract, cooperation, and the importance of money and power in all human affairs. She thinks that what gives her a right to "treat" her "mad" patients is her professional training and license, not the patients' desire for help, consent to treatment, and willingness to pay for it.

An ardent feminist, Ussher believes that madness in females is caused by males. In pretentious, deconstructionist-socialist prose, she declares, "'Madness' acts as a signifier which positions women as ill, as outside, as pathological, as somehow second-rate—the second sex."[57] Nevertheless, she uses the language of psychopathology and goes out of her way—perhaps in an effort to further establish her professional *bona fides* as a clinical psychologist—to criticize my advocating the abolition of psychiatric coercion. In a section revealingly titled "The negation of reality," Ussher states: "Szasz's image of the forcibly incarcerated victim was never a reality for those deemed mad in recent years."[58] This is a breathtakingly untruthful assertion. Psychiatric practices in Australia, Canada, Britain, and the United States closely resemble one another. The Australian Mental Health Act of 1993—similar to mental health legislation in the United Kingdom and the United States—contains a section entitled, "Orders for admission and detention."[59] So much for psychiatric incarceration never being a "reality" in Australia after 1970.

Ussher continues: "Today it is more likely that people are desperately hanging on with the hope of some salvation, whilst the waiting list of the psychiatrist or psychologist on which they have placed themselves recedes slowly in front of them."[60] "Waiting list"? Ussher is a true child of the therapeutic state in which consensual psychotherapeutic relationships are regarded as exploitative and evil and are accordingly "prohibited."[61] The only morally correct "mental health service" is a public service, funded by the government, with "services" being provided by agents of the state.[62] Denying that mental health services rest on coercion, Ussher condemns "the dissenters...[who] profit from the rhetoric, from the critiques, but they do not want to dirty their hands with the real questions: What to do about madness? What to say to those *who demand help*?"[63]

Patients with cancer and diabetes do not *demand* help. Polite persons do not *demand* goods and services, especially not from strangers; they ask, request, seek, suggest, and offer payment or services or at least gratitude for what they receive, often before receiving it. In the world of private exchanges, no one is entitled to anything. The answer to Ussher's question, "What to say to those *who demand help*?" is, "Grow up and learn some manners!" Ussher patronizes the "consumers of mental health services": Like wailing infants, they have the "right" to make demands, even on strangers, and they have a "right" to the satisfaction of their demands.

Ussher is an enthusiast for a pharmacratic-psychiatric totalitarian political system the principal function of which is to service "madwomen." In a section titled, "Re-educating the experts," she explains: "This [overthrowing 'the law of the phallus'] does not remove from the professionals the onus to change.... Just as the academic deconstruction needs to be interdisciplinary, so must the professional intervention. A woman may *need* economic support, child care, psychotropic medication or therapy." Ussher's "madwoman" has only needs; she has no responsibilities.

Ussher approvingly cites my statement in *The Manufacture of Madness*, "The concept of mental illness has the same logical and empirical status as the concept of witchcraft."[64] However, she fails to recognize that my comment implies that mental illness does not "exist." Only after belief in the existence of witches was thoroughly discredited did the persecution of witches end. *Mutatis mutandis*, only after belief in the existence of mental illness is thoroughly discredited—and only after psychiatric inquisitors (a.k.a. mental health/illness professionals) disappear from the social scene—will we be in a position to begin to really help the vast numbers of diverse individuals we call "mentally ill."

Ussher's views about Virginia Woolf are driven by her feminist and "health psychologist" zeal and are unrelated to the facts about Woolf: "Virginia Woolf eloquently describes what she sees as woman's eternal role—the mirror for man's glory. She is always second best, always the second sex. If this is so, it is no wonder that women are mad.... Women are significantly poorer than men."[65] Virginia was not a mirror for Leonard's glory, nor was she poorer than her husband. Vita Sackville-West was not a mirror to her husband's, Harold Nicolson's, glory. Virginia Woolf never said that a woman's role is to be a mirror for a man's glory. She said that she lived in a male-dominated society, which was correct and obvious. Women still live in a male-dominated society and are, in general, poorer than men. Every group, every society, is hierarchical. If subordination to a superior made subordinates go mad, then virtually everyone would be mad. Ussher, however, systematically attributes "women's madness" to men. She does not tell us what causes "men's madness." She concludes: "There can be no simple answer to the question of whether women's madness is a misogynistic construct, or a mental illness."[66] Ussher goes to a lot of trouble showing what men have always known: that women drive them crazy.[67]

Appendix II

The Mad Genius Problem

1

Our ideas about genius, madness, and the existence of a close relationship between them are modern inventions. For millennia, people explained the world about them—especially creative-good and destructive-bad behaviors—in spiritual or God terms.

In the biblical view, creativity is the prerogative of a single supreme Creator. The Scripture attributes the miracle of life to a specific divine act, God's literally "breathing life" into Adam's nostrils: "And the Lord God formed man of the dust of the ground, and breathed into his nostrils the breath of life; and man became living soul" (Genesis, 2:7). Hence comes our notion of *inspiration* as an explanation for great works of art and science. The idea of "inspiration"—of breath, soul, or some other mysterious "substance" entering the person from without and enabling him to perform exceptionally good or bad deeds—has never lost its influence on western thought. It is the source of the notion of possession (by spirits), and its modern successors, "possession" by the *creative inspiration* of genius and by the *destructive irresistible impulse* of madness. We replace spirit-God words with body-mind words and exult in our smug conviction that we are explaining exceptionally good and bad behaviors scientifically.

The term "genius" comes from the Latin *gignere*, meaning to beget. In the Roman world, every person was attended by a tutelary deity or spirit, his *genius*. The Latin *inspirare*, from *in* + *spirare*, to breathe, meant to influence, move, or guide by divine or supernatural inspiration. None of these notions had anything to do with illness or mental illness in the modern sense. Nevertheless, to buttress the cause of psychiatry, psychiatrists cite the views of famous ancients

115

on the connections between genius and madness—for example, Aristotle's statement, "No great genius has ever existed without some touch of madness," or Seneca's remark, "There is no great genius without some touch of madness." Aristotle and Seneca were saying that both the genius and the madman are *inspired by spirits more powerful than those that inspire ordinary persons*. They did not mean that genius and madness are biological conditions, or medical diseases, or the manifestations of diseases.

In fact, when Aristotle and Seneca and other Greek and Roman philosophers offered pronouncements about genius and madness, they uttered tautologies that sounded, and perhaps still sound, like deep insights: They stated that persons who performed exceptional deeds were exceptionally inspired persons. The pseudoscience of psychiatry has, in effect, replaced *spirits possessing the person* as an explanation for his *devilish mind*, with *chemical processes in the brain* as an explanation for his *diseased mind*. The ancients believed in spirits: They were not empiricists and needed no evidence of the material existence of spirits. We moderns are "scientific" and demand empirical "proof" for medical explanations. In the absence of objective evidence for the claim that brain chemicals cause creativity-genius and crime-madness, psychiatrists and science writers use the testimonials of celebrities to support their claim. The confessionals of the writer William Styron, television journalist Mike Wallace, and psychologist Kay Redfield Jamison are typical. This strategy for supporting the physical existence/material reality of mental illnesses leads to some bizarre outcomes.

For example, Anthony Storr—a respected British psychiatrist and Jungian analyst—declares: "We owe an immense debt to the many men and women of genius who have suffered from manic-depressive illness."[1] Debt for what? For the pleasure and wisdom their creations have brought us? Certainly. For having suffered from manic-depressive illness? Certainly not. We are not expected to feel indebted to men and women of genius for having suffered from syphilis or tuberculosis, diseases that formerly afflicted many such persons.

Moreover, it is not enough that we are asked to believe that there is some sort of special connection between manic-depression and creativity, we are also asked to believe that that imaginary connection obligates the "patient-genius" to be grateful to his disease, and the public to be grateful to the "suffering patient." There is no scientific evidence to support this romantic-depressing-medical image of the mad genius. It is sustained, instead, partly by great performances by fine actors in didactic films, such as *The Hours*, and largely by government agencies and psychiatric propaganda.

Alongside the romantic image of manic-depression as a cause of creativity that does not detract from the subject's intentionality for his conduct and responsibility for his good deeds stands the bleak image of schizophrenia as a cause of criminality annulling the subject's intentionality for his conduct and responsibility for his bad deeds. This interpretation, too, lacks objective proof. Instead, its "truth" is enshrined in, and is taught by, the modern clerical and clinical practices of the insanity excuse/defense. Clergymen of all denominations now bury *all* persons who break the religious law against self-killing in consecrated ground, "diagnosing" all suicides automatically *non compos mentis* at the precise moment of their sinful deed. Similarly, the insanity defense allows lawyers, judges, psychiatrists, and society to incarcerate *some* persons who break secular laws in prisons called "hospitals," "diagnosing" all such criminals as having been *non compos mentis* at the precise moment of their illegal action.[2]

2

The second half of the eighteenth century ushered in revolutionary changes in scientific, social, and political thought. The writings of the French philosophes; the founding of the United States; the publication of Adam Smith's *The Wealth of Nations*; the French Revolution; the establishment of the profession of mad-doctoring, madness as a disease of the brain, genius as a "faculty" located in the brain—all these events and ideas have their origins in that period.

A Treatise on Madness by William Battie, the first modern medical text on madness by a physician, was published in 1758. In 1774, the English "Madhouse Act" for the regulation of private madhouses became law. The same year, the Scottish philosopher Alexander Gerard published his *Essay on Genius.* Gerard invented the idea that man possesses a "faculty of invention" by means of which he becomes "qualified for making new discoveries in science or for producing original works of art."[3] In 1788, King George III—who suffered from porphyria, a metabolic disease with central nervous system symptoms—was "treated" by mad-doctors.

In his study, *The Mad Genius Controversy*, sociologist George Becker traces the development of the idea that madness and genius are closely related and demonstrates many of its weaknesses. While much of the material he presents is useful, many of his observations and conclusions are inaccurate. I agree that "It is around the start of the eighteenth century that the term genius began to acquire its modern meaning, in the sense that it was used to denote a mysterious quality—a creative energy—that certain individuals were assessed as possessing."[4] But I do not agree that "The stereotype of the mad genius reached its apex of popularity at the turn of the twentieth century (1880-1920). It has been largely discredited during the post-World War II period—at least in academic circles...one can place the development of the concept of the mad genius firmly in the period between 1836 and 1950."[5] The evidence presented in this book and the vast contemporary literature on the subject of the mad genius flatly contradict this conclusion.[6] Belief in the notions of genius and madness not merely as concepts but as identifiable entities or qualities (in the brain), and in a demonstrable connection between them, is more firmly and more widely held today than at any time in the past.

For example, Kay Redfield Jamison, a psychologist with a personal and professional axe to grind, and Clifford A. Pickover, a science writer dazzled by neuroscience, are equally convinced of the reality of the "mad genius." The subtitle of Pickover's popular book, *Strange Brains and Genius: The Secret Lives of Eccentric Scientists and Madmen*, is misleading.[7] "And" in the title implies that the author studied both scientists *and* madmen, which is not the case. Pickering begins with the premise that creative people ("geniuses") tend to be mad and proves it by documenting the eccentricities of many creative people. The jacket blurb states: "Clifford Pickover, internationally recognized science popularizer...delights us with unexpected stories of their [the mad scientists'] obsessive personalities and strange phobias. These common threads lead us to wonder if creativity and genius are inextricably linked to madness."

The book received rave reviews. *Publisher's Weekly* praised it: "Filled with 200 years of eccentric geniuses, this delightful collection of profiles assembles an eclectic and fascinating sampling of scientists (as well as some artists and writers) with a far-ranging assortment of phobias, compulsions, odd belief systems and extraordinarily weird habits." The reviewer for the *New Scientist* embraced the thesis: "Clifford Pickover in *Strange Brains and Genius* provides more than enough evidence to show that an astounding intellect can be a passport to insanity.... What is the connection between genius and madness? IBM-based polymath Clifford Pickover...looks at the lives of a collection of eccentric scientists, from Nikolai Tesla to the Unabomber, giving each a name ('The Fly Man from Galway'; 'The Rat Man from London') deliberately reminiscent of Sigmund Freud's names for his cases. Then Pickover discusses obsessive-compulsive disorder and the relationship between brain structure and genius."

As recently as 1992, James Gleick titled his biography of Richard Feynman *Genius*, adding *The Life and Science of Richard Feynman* as a subtitle. At the same time, with the astuteness and honesty characteristic of his writing, Gleick acknowledged that the term "genius" is virtually meaningless, an evocative expression of high praise, not a description of anything identifiable, objectifiable, measurable, or falsifiable:

> What a strange and bewildering literature grew up around the term genius—defining it, analyzing it, categorizing it, rationalizing and reifying it. Commentators have contrasted it with such qualities as (mere) talent, intellect, imagination, originality, industriousness, sweep of mind and elegance of style.... Psychologists and philosophers, musicologists and art critics, historians of science and scientists themselves have all stepped into this quagmire, a capacious one. Their centuries of labor have produced no consensus on any of the necessary questions. Is there such a quality? If so, where does it come from?... When otherwise sober scientists speak of the genius as magician, wizard, or superhuman, are they merely indulging in a flight of literary fancy?... And a question that has barely been asked...: Why, as the pool of available humans has risen from one hundred million to one billion to five billion, has the production of geniuses—Shakespeares, Newtons, Mozarts, Einsteins—seemingly choked off to nothing, genius itself coming to seem like the property of the past?[8]

We also ought to ask, paraphrasing Gleick: With life so much longer and healthier than in the past, why is the "production of madmen and madwomen" coming to seem like a property of the present? The answers to these questions lie in a more critical understanding of cultural history and the uses of language, not in research in neuroscience or propaganda for psychopharmacology. Mockingly, Gleick asks: "When people speak of the borderline between genius and madness, why is it so evident what they mean?" In the same mocking spirit, I venture to answer: Because that is how they can earn glowing reviews in the media for their books on neuromythology and receive lucrative "genius awards" from the MacArthur Foundation.[9]

3

The belief that research in neuroscience and psychiatry will "explain" the alleged connection between genius and madness is a typically modern delusion. Almost a hundred years ago, the great German psychiatrist Ernst Kretscher (1888-1964) acknowledged that the notion of "mad genius" is a psychiatric invention: "Since the Italian alienist, [Cesare] Lombroso, first coined that pregnant expression 'genius and madness' there has arisen in educated circles a very lively discussion, which, however, has been forced to close with the recognition that modern psychiatry has been responsible for—some might say guilty of—establishing such a connection."[10]

Genius and madness are vague terms. The only thing clear about them is that, by definition, each term refers to a type of psychological abnormality, *a deviation from a behavioral-social norm.* Genius and madness are value terms, not medical or scientific terms. One is deviation up (good) and is rewarded; the other is deviation down (bad) and is punished.

In its contemporary use, then, the term "genius" simply means being very good at something—whether it is mathematics or music, ballet or botany, curing or killing. Being exceptionally virtuous and being exceptionally wicked both count as genius. Stalin and Hitler were geniuses: They excelled in mass-producing corpses, just as Henry Ford excelled in mass-producing cars.

The modern meaning of genius as (hereditary) excellence was shaped largely by Sir Francis Galton (1822-1911), the father of eugenics. Galton was born into a wealthy and distinguished Quaker family: Erasmus Darwin, a famous physician and botanist, was his maternal grandfather. Charles Darwin was his cousin. "Darwin had thought mainly about the evolution of physical features, like wings and eyes," observes science writer Jim Holt. Applying the same hereditary logic to mental attributes, like talent and virtue, Galton lamented: "If a twentieth part of the cost and pains were spent in measures for the improvement of the human race that is spent on the improvements of the breed of horses and cattle, what a galaxy of genius might we not create!"[11]

How did Galton know that genius is hereditary? The same way that, imitating Galton, the modern psychiatrist knows that manic-depression is hereditary.[12] "In his 1869 book *Hereditary Genius*, Galton "assembled long lists of 'eminent' men—judges, poets, scientists, even oarsmen and wrestlers—to show that excellence ran in families."[13]

A cow produces prodigious quantities of milk: She is a bovine genius. A man paints beautiful pictures: He is an artistic genius. Einstein is a scientific genius. Mozart is a musical genius. Are Abraham, Moses, Jesus, and Mohammed religious geniuses? Are we explaining achievement when we attribute it to the fictitious entity we call "genius," or are we deceiving ourselves the same way that the scientifically unsophisticated person deceives himself when he declares that hydrogen burns because it is "flammable"?

It is true that breeders of animals can produce cows that give lots of milk and horses that win races. The breeder decides, the animal (re)produces. People already do something like this. Men and women choose mates with whom to have children, and bring up children to cultivate the skills (traits) that they, the parents, value. The child can no more choose his parents than the horse can choose its owner-breeder. But the child soon gains power—both physical and legal-political—to cultivate the traits he values, and reject the traits he disvalues. Doing so, he often displeases his breeders, his parents.

What kinds of persons would a breeder of humans want to produce? Obviously, the answer depends on the values and goals of the individual who controls the breeding. Galton wanted to breed a race of persons resembling himself, "creative geniuses." Ironically, the Galtons had no children. He or his wife was sterile. Galton was said to have suffered two "nervous breakdowns." Was he a mad genius?

The two great twentieth century dictators both fancied themselves geneticists. Stalin personally elevated Trofim Lysenko to the status of genius and made him, in 1928, the genetics czar of the Soviet Union. Lysenkoism became a campaign against genetics and geneticists: Scientific genetics was stigmatized as a "fascist science" and the leading geneticists were executed or exiled. The term survives as a metaphor for false beliefs, refuted by empirical evidence but preferred for ideological reasons.[14] Persuaded by the Marxist-Leninist ideology that breeding a "new Socialist man" was a task for politics not biology, Stalin was not interested in using eugenics as a political tool.

Hitler, in contrast, went all the way politicizing Galtonian eugenics. He too sought to improve the "human stock." The genius he admired was martial and misogynist: Men should be warriors, women should be mothers, and all should be members of the "Aryan race."[15] Accordingly, Hitler sought to breed "healthy" Aryans and eliminate "racial degenerates," such as Jews, Gypsies, homosexuals, and the mentally ill.

4

The name of the Italian psychiatrist Cesare Lombroso (1835-1909) is all but forgotten today. Born thirteen years after Francis Galton and twenty-one years before Freud, Lombroso was the first "Darwinian-eugenicist" psychiatrist: He combined evolution, medicine, moral judgment, law, and criminal punishment to rationalize and justify the therapeutic state, with the psychiatrist as philosopher-king. "Genius," he declared, "is one of the many forms of insanity."[16] Criminality was also a form of insanity. Ordinary insanity was also insanity. These discoveries made him one of the most famous scientists of his age.

In 1872—only three years after the appearance of Galton's *Hereditary Genius*—Lombroso published *Genius and Madness* (*Genio e Follia*), the book that launched his fame. According to Lombroso, genius is closely allied with madness, the two "conditions" forming two faces of the same psychobiological reality. Italian psychiatrists Giuseppe Carrà and Francesco Barale explain: "[Lombroso] stated that a man of genius was essentially a degenerate whose 'madness' was a form of evolutionary compensation for excessive intellectual development."

Recognizing the publicity value of the evolutionary-hereditary model, Lombroso is an unrecognized pioneer of the currently fashionable evolutionary psychology. In 1876, he published *The Criminal Man* (*L'uomo Delinquente*), the book that made him a very famous man. Carrà and Barale write: "In this work, Lombroso employed Darwinian ideas of evolution to account for criminal behavior.... [He held] that there is a degenerate class of human beings, distinguished by anatomical and psychical characteristics, who are born with criminal instincts and who represent a reversion to a very primitive form of humanity."[17]

The life and work of Ernst Kretschmer form a bridge between the Galton-Lombroso-Freud era and our post-World War II era of neo-

Kraepelinian, mental illness-is-brain-disease imperial psychiatry. Kretschmer's thinking was heavily influenced by Lombroso's work and he shared the deep-seated psychiatric-eugenic belief that madness (genius) is a hereditary disease, a genetic curse. He wrote: "The fate which hangs over the family of the man of genius is part of the deepest tragedy of these strange personalities."[18] Although Kretschmer recognized that the notion of the mad genius was a product manufactured by psychiatry, and that the terms "genius" and "mad" are value terms, he was not prepared to impede his profession's rapidly increasing prestige, influence, and growth. Treating genius and madness as if they were medical terms, Kretschmer complained: "Why now does one run against such powerful opposition when one asserts this fact?" His answer was: "Largely owing to the prejudice of 'psychopathic inferiority'; the opinion that the mentally sound are always superior to the less spiritually normal, not only in a biological, but also in a social, sense.... So we may conclude that psychopaths and the mentally diseased play a most important part in the development of national life, a role which might be graphically compared to that of the microbe in other organisms."[19] Only a few years later, German psychiatrists took the analogy literally and drew the logical conclusion that the madman, like the microbe, needed to be destroyed by poison gas. However, it must be noted that Kretschmer was one of the psychiatrists in Nazi Germany who took no part in the extermination of mental patients.

Kretschmer's *The Psychology of Men of Genius* was translated into English by Raymond Bernard Cattell (1905-1998), who later became one of the most prominent psychologists in the English-speaking world. In his "Translator's Foreword," Cattell wrote : "[T]he real, scientific study of this *biological problem* began with the modern psychological researches of Dr. Lombroso and Sir Francis Galton."[20] Note that Cattell, like Kretschmer, treats genius as a "biological problem," and psychology as a biological science. Still, in his Foreword, Cattell criticized Kretschmer, for example, for the absurdly misogynous view that there can be no women geniuses because "every woman genius is so because at heart she is a man."[21] Cattell also offered some astute observations, for example, that "those who write of genius and compile National Biographies always give such a huge representation to literary and artistic men, and leave out great business organizers, engineers, etc. Possibly they feel that the latter already have their reward in the salaries that they command."[22]

The possibly unintended wittiness of this remark dispels, at least momentarily, the dreary pretentiousness of the pseudoscience of the mad-genius research. In my view, the Galton-Lombroso-Kretschmer premise—really, one ought to say bias—treats both genius and madness as abnormal biological conditions and thus precludes intelligent investigation and humane understanding of both exceptional achievement ("genius") and exceptional failure ("madness").

Edison knew neither genetics nor psychology, but he knew what genius was firsthand. It was, he said, "one per cent inspiration and ninety-nine per cent perspiration."

5

Not surprisingly, the supposed connections between genius and madness have generated, and continue to generate, vast quantities of pretentious nonsense. In part this is because both terms masquerade as descriptions but function as injunctions: One exalts and glorifies the subject, the other debases and demonizes him. Genius implies good; mad implies bad. The creator-genius and destroyer-madman resemble one another in their single-minded determination to achieve their goal.

Nineteenth-century French alienists medicalized single-mindedness by calling it "monomania." According to the *Oxford English Dictionary*, the term, first used in 1823, refers to "A form of insanity in which the patient is irrational on one subject only"; it is also used to identify "An exaggerated enthusiasm for or devotion to one subject; a craze." In different times and in different places people value devotion to a particular subject differently. This simple fact explains why certain persons dishonored as mad at one time may later be hailed as geniuses, and vice versa. While he was alive, the Hungarian obstetrician, Ignaz Semmelweis—who discovered the microbial etiology of puerperal fever before the discovery of the pathogenic role of microbes—was considered to possess an erroneous belief, which he defended with "irrational" intensity. Diagnosed insane, he was incarcerated and died in a madhouse. Today, the medical school at the University of Budapest is named after him. Conversely, while he was alive, Adolf Hitler was hailed, especially by Germans while he was victorious, as a political and military genius. Today, he is loathed as a lunatic.

Our images of the genius and the madman resemble each other in that we perceive both as persons so powerfully possessed by an interest that they appear to be under the control of an alien power—a "muse" in antiquity, "genius" and "madness" today. The connection between genius and madness is an artifact, not a biological or medical condition or phenomenon. The two "images" stand in the same sort of relation to one another as do the negative and positive images of a photograph (taken in the predigital age of photography).

We view both the genius and the mad person as "inspired." However, "science tells us to regard the former as *intentionality incarnate*, and the latter as *devoid of intentionality*; the good genius (great artist) as possessing moral agency and personal responsibility, and the bad genius (mad criminal) as bereft of these quintessentially human qualities. These constructions suit our needs for dealing with persons who exhibit exceptional conduct. They are not scientifically valid accounts of a person's *ability to control his behavior.* Persons called "creative" or "crazy" or both are capable of self-control; each yields to his inclinations, whose consequences others judge to be good ("creative") or bad ("crazy"). The doctrine that the so-called insane person *cannot* control his behavior is a factually unsupported postulate parading as a factual proposition. Although everyone's behavior is manifestly intentional, we split people into three groups: individuals with exceptionally large amounts of intentionality, the geniuses; those with an average amount of intentionality, ordinary, normal persons; and those with little or no intentionality, the insane.

We regard the genius as full of intentionality: His creative act is the embodiment of self-disciplined self-expression. We equate the actor with his act. For example, we say about a painting by Renoir: "It is a Renoir."

We regard the madman as lacking intentionality: His destructive act is the embodiment of alienated impulsivity. We separate the actor from his act. For example, we say about an insane murderer: "He was not himself."

Our ideas about absent intentionality and annulled responsibility and the policies based on them—for example, the insanity defense and tort litigation for voluntary behavior, such as smoking—are artifacts, the consequences of our belief in mental illness. The answer to the question, "Was Virginia Woolf a genius or a mad woman or a mad genius?" tells us more about the speaker than it does about Virginia Woolf.

6

One of the cardinal characteristics of the true genius is that—like Jesus on the cross—he *suffers* (inter alia, from madness). This belief, like all religious belief, is impervious to empirical evidence; its specialized language is its own proof. The Internet biography of the Norwegian artist Edvard Munch is illustrative. His work, we are informed, "symbolize[s] the tortured genius who must pay for his creativity with madness and misery.... The artist's brooding, anguished and powerful work, [was] based on personal grief and obsessions."[23]

The genius who does not suffer cannot be a true genius. The happy genius is an oxymoron. Examples to the contrary are brushed away. Peter Paul Rubens (1577-1640), one of the greatest painters of all time, had a normal childhood, was a competent, worldly person who spoke five languages, was financially successful, and was never considered insane.[24] "Given the magnificence of his success," writes Peter Schjeldahl, art critic for the *New Yorker*, "there's little wonder that he lacked the shadier, more refractory genius of a Caravaggio, a Rembrandt, or a Velasquez. *He was too happy*."[25] Hence, Rubens does not qualify as a genius.

Einstein lived a "normal," "happy" life. Never mind. Explains the British Broadcasting Company: "Einstein has become an icon of science universally recognized the world over but beyond the cliché of the mad genius lay, well, a mad genius—who hated socks."[26]

Unfortunately, many of the cleverest and most memorable aphorisms about genius and madness are simply dead wrong. "When a true genius appears in the world," Samuel Johnson famously observed, "you may know him by this sign: that all the dunces are in confederacy against him." The appearance in the world of Newton, Faraday, Edison, Planck, Einstein, Feynman, and other geniuses, especially in the hard sciences, prove Johnson wrong.

Notes

Epigraph

1. Oates, J. C., "The Art of Suicide," in Donnelly, J., ed., *Suicide: Right or Wrong?* (Buffalo: Prometheus Books, 1990), pp. 207-212; p. 212.

Preface

1. Snyder, Allan W. "Genius, Madness, and Innovation," ATSE Focus No 125, January/February 2003, http://www.atse.org.au/index.php?sectionid=492. A mathematician, physicist, and renowned researcher in vision, Snyder is one of Australia's most honored and famous scientists: He is a fellow of the Royal Society of London and the society's 2001 Clifford Paterson Prize Lecturer; the recipient of the Marconi International Prize, recognized as the world's foremost prize in communication and information technology, in 2001; and of the Australia Prize, 1997.

2. Caines, M., "Reflections of Iris," *TLS*, February 15, 2004, p. 15.

3. Ingram, M., "Virginia Woolf's psychiatric history," June 2002. http://ourworld.compuserve.com/homepages/malcolmi/; see also, http://www.rcpsych.ac.uk/info/webguide/psychobio.htm. Virginia has also been diagnosed as schizophrenic: "Virginia Woolf's novels represent many aspects of early schizophrenia. The hermit-like isolation and refusal to interact on a deeper personal level, as seen in Woolf's *To the Lighthouse*, are clear symptoms of early stages of schizophrenia."

4. Bergemann, M., "Insanity in Modern Literature," http://www.holycross.edu/departments/english/preynold/Insanity_and_Literature.html.

5. For example, see "Native American convert to Catholicism, declared as 'blessed' and a candidate for sainthood: Kateri Tekawitha (1656-1680)," http://demo.lutherproductions.com/historytutor/basic/modern/people/tekawitha.htm. Converted to Catholicism, Tekawitha ended up in Montreal, where "she became spiritually devoted to the Virgin Mary and practiced many forms of self-denial. After her death at age 24, miraculous cures were attributed to her.... In 1980 she was beatified or declared to have attained blessedness. She is a candidate for sainthood, the first Native American and the first American laywoman to be so honored."

6. Szasz, T., "The Uses of Naming and the Origin of the Myth of Mental Illness," *American Psychologist*, 16: 59-65 (February), 1961, reprinted as "The Rhetoric of Rejection," in *Ideology and Insanity: Essays on the Psychiatric Dehumanization of Man* [1970] (Syracuse: Syracuse University Press, 1991), pp. 49-68; and *The Myth of Mental Illness: Foundations of a Theory of Personal Conduct* [1961]. Revised edition (New York: HarperCollins, 1974).

7. Shakespeare, W., *As You Like It*, Act 2, Scene 7, lines 139-167.

8. Ingram, http://ourworld.compuserve.com/homepages/malcolmi/attacks2.htm.

9. Jones, E., *The Life and Work of Sigmund Freud* (3 vols.; New York: Basic Books, 1953-1957), vol. 3, p. 45, emphasis added.

10.   Szasz, T., *The Therapeutic State: Psychiatry in the Mirror of Current Events* (Buffalo: Prometheus Books, 1984).

11.   Edlin, G., quoted in Magnus, D., "The Concept of Genetic Disease," in Caplan, A. L., McCartney, J. J., and Sisti, D. A., eds., *Health, Disease, and Illness: Concepts in Medicine* (Washington, D.C.: Georgetown University Press, 2004), pp. 233-242; pp. 238, 240.

12.   Magnus, D., "The Concept of Genetic Disease," ibid.

13.   Goffman, E. *Asylums: Essays on the Social Situation of Mental Patients and Other Inmates* (Garden City, NY: Doubleday Anchor, 1961), pp. 135, 137-138.

14.   Ibid., p. 379.

15.   Faulkner, W., *As I Lay Dying* [1930] (New York: Vintage Books/Random House, 1957), p. 223.

16.   Bleuler, E., *Dementia Praecox or the Group of Schizophrenias* [1911]. Translated by Joseph Zinkin (New York: International Universities Press, 1950), p. 327.

17.   Szasz, T., *The Myth of Mental Illness: Foundations of a Theory of Personal Conduct* (New York: Paul B. Hoeber, 1961); revised edition (New York: HarperCollins, 1974).

18.   Kretschmer, E., *Hysteria, Reflex, and Instinct* [1923] (New York: Philosophical Library, 1960), p. 68.

19.   In modern (pseudo-) egalitarian societies, the role of power in human relations tends to be denied, especially by the powerful, nowhere more than in psychiatry: (Nominally) the rule is, "What's sauce for the goose is sauce for the gander." Psychiatrists, patients, and the family are all entitled to diagnose disease.

20.   See Sadler, J. C. and Fulford B., "Should patients and their families contribute to the DSM-V process?" *Psychiatric Services*, 2004; 55: 133-138; Szasz, T., "Malingering: 'Diagnosis' or social condemnation?" *A.M.A. Archives of Neurology and Psychiatry*, 76: 432-443 (October), 1956; "What is malingering?" *Medical Trial Technique Quarterly*, 6: 29-40 (September), 1959; *The Myth of Mental Illness*, op. cit.; and "'Idiots, infants, and the insane': Mental Illness and legal incompetence," *Journal of Medical Ethics*, 31: 78-81 (February), 2005. http://jme.bmjjournals.com/cgi/content/abstract/ 31/2/78?etoc.

21.   Szasz, T., *The Myth of Mental Illness*, op. cit.

22.   Kretschmer, E., *Hysteria, Reflex, and Instinct*, op. cit., p. 69, emphasis added.

23.   Ibid., pp. 69, 91.

24.   Szasz, T., *Pharmacracy: Medicine and Politics in America* [2001] (Syracuse: Syracuse University Press, 2003).

25.   Mann, T., *Confessions of Felix Krull, Confidence Man* [1954]. Translated by Denver Lindley (New York: Signet/New American Library, 1957).

26.   Rosenhan, D. L., "On being sane in insane places," *Science*, 179: 250258 (January), 1973.

27.   "Who is the Gipper from the saying, 'one for the Gipper?'," http://www.clockguy.com/PreviewStoryBoards.html. George Gipp, "the Gipper," was born in 1895. From 1917 to 1920, he was a varsity athlete at the University of Notre Dame. While planning to pursue a career in baseball, he was convinced by legendary college coach Knute Rockne to play football as well. He led the Fighting Irish to a 27-2-3 record. During one of his final football games at Notre Dame, Gipp caught a throat infection and died a few weeks later at the age of twenty-five. Just before his death, he told Coach Rockne, "Some time, Rock, when the team is up against it, when things are wrong and the breaks are beating the boys—tell them to go in there with all they've got and win just one for the Gipper. I don't know where I'll be then, Rock. But I'll know about it, and I'll be happy."

Chapter 1. "Whatever we are to call it"

1. The British government paid compensation to slave owners, the amount depending on the number of slaves. For example, "the Bishop of Exeter's 665 slaves resulted in him receiving £12,700, an enormous sum at that time." See "1833 Abolition of Slavery Act," http://www.spartacus.schoolnet.co.uk/Lslavery33.htm.

2. "Sir Leslie Stephen, " *Dictionary of National Biography*, Oxford University Press, http://www.oup.com/oxforddnb/info/about/dictionary/history/lsbiog.html. Eton was, and still is, one of the most exclusive schools in England.

3. In Virginia's day, upper-class women no longer had "spells." She and her family typically referred to her periods of despair, dependence on others, and aggressive behavior as "breakdowns" or as "going mad." The entry for Virginia Woolf in the *Dictionary of National Biography* uses the latter term. http://www.archiveshub.ac.uk/news/vlwoolf.html.

4. Bell, Q., *Virginia Woolf*, vol. 1, p. 44, emphasis added.

5. Ibid.

6. Ibid., p. 90.

7. King, J., *Virginia Woolf* (New York: Norton, 1994), pp. 33-34.

8. Bell, Q., *Virginia Woolf*, vol. 1, p. 89.

9. Quoted in Poole, R., *The Unknown Virginia Woolf* (Cambridge: Cambridge University Press, 1978), p. 40.

10. Quoted in Spater, G. and Parsons, I., *A Marriage of True Minds: An Intimate Portrait of Leonard and Virginia Woolf* (New York: Harcourt Brace Jovanovich, 1977), p. 58.

11. Woolf, V., *Letters*, vol. 1, p. 615.

12. Ibid.

13. Quoted in, Skidelsky, R., *John Maynard Keynes: Volume One, Hopes Betrayed, 1883-1920* (New York: Viking, 1986), p. xxvi.

14. Auden, W. H., *The Dyer's Hand, and Other Essays* [1962] (New York: Vintage, 1968), p. 14.

15. Spater, G., and Parsons, I., *A Marriage of True Minds*, op. cit.

16. Bell, Q., *Virginia Woolf*, vol. 2, p. 5.

17. Ibid.

18. Burke, E., "Jacobinism," in Bredvold, L. T. and Ross, R. G., editors, *The Philosophy of Edmund Burke, A Selection from his Speeches and Writings* (Ann Arbor, MI: University of Michigan Press, 1960), p. 249.

19. Bell, Q., *Virginia Woolf*, vol. 2, p. 6.

20. Quoted in ibid.

21. Ibid., p. 7.

22. Ibid.

23. Ibid. It is not clear whether Savage offered this opinion in Virginia's presence or, if not, whether she was informed of it.

24. Sir Maurice Craig (1866-1935) was a fashionable specialist in "nervous diseases," with the largest consulting practice of his time. He also owned and ran a "nursing home," and was the author of *Psychological Medicine: A Manual on Mental Disease for Practitioners and Students* [1905] (Philadelphia: P. Blakiston's Son & Co., 1917).

25. Theophilus Bulkeley Hyslop (1863-1933) was a prominent English psychiatrist. His publications include *Mental Physiology: Especially in Its Relations to Mental Disorders* (Philadelphia: P. Blakiston, Son & Co., 1895), *The Great Abnormals* (London: P. Allan, 1925), and *Mental Handicaps in Golf* (London: Bailliere, Tindall & Cox, 1927).

26.   Bell, Q., *Virginia Woolf*, vol. 2, p. 8.
27.   Ibid.
28.   The need to love, if acknowledged at all, is astonishingly neglected in psychology and psychoanalysis. Margot Fonteyn (1919-1991), the legendary English ballerina, sensitively acknowledged that she married because of her need to love: "I so much wanted to love and it seemed so difficult for me to love...my need to love far outweighed my need to be loved." Quoted in Gottlieb, R., "The art of pleasing," *New York Review of Books*, December 2, 2004, pp. 15-17; p. 15.
29.   Woolf, L., *Beginning Again: An Autobiography of the Years 1911-1918* (New York: Harcourt, Brace & World, 1964), p. 155. Sir Henry Head (1861-1940), a prominent neurologist, was a famously arrogant, domineering, know-it-all kind of physician. "One day the bacteriologist William Bulloch (1868-1941) asked him over lunch at his hospital whether he had read Hagenheimer's new book on locomotor ataxia. Head replied he had only had time to glance at it. Bullock commented, 'Well, you have done better than the rest of us. There is no such book.'" http://www.whonamedit.\com/doctor.cfm/705.html.
30.   Ibid., p., 156, emphasis added.
31.   As I noted earlier, it is not clear whether Virginia was aware of this recommendation.
32.   Woolf, L., *Beginning Again*, op. cit., p. 156.
33.   Ibid.
34.   Malcolm Ingram's Homepage, "Virginia Woolf's Psychiatric History: 1913-1914: A Major Attack and Suicidal Attempt," http://ourworld.compuserve.com/homepages/malcolmi/attacks2.htm. 2000.
35.   Woolf, L., *Beginning Again*, op. cit., p. 159.
36.   Bell, Q., *Virginia Woolf*, vol. 2, p. 12.

Chapter 2. "In the head you know"

1.   Szasz, T., editor, *The Age of Madness: A History of Involuntary Mental Hospitalization Presented in Selected Texts* (Garden City, NY: Doubleday Anchor, 1973).
2.   Szasz, T., *The Manufacture of Madness: A Comparative Study of the Inquisition and the Mental Health Movement* [1970] (Syracuse: Syracuse University Press, 1997).
3.   Mitchell, L., *Bulwer Lytton: The Rise and Fall of a Victorian Man of Letters* (London: Hambledon & London, 2003).
4.   "Dysfunctional to a spectacular degree," 29/06/2003. http://www.telegraph.co.uk/arts/main.jhtml?xml=/arts/2003/06/29/bomit22.xml.
5.   http://www.litencyc.com/php/speople.php?rec=true&UID=637
6.   Lytton, R. B., *A Blighted Life: A True Story* [1880] (Bristol, UK: Thoemmes Press, 1994).
7.   Gilman, C. P., *The Yellow Wallpaper* [1892]. Edited by Dale M. Bauer (Boston: Bedford/St. Martin's, 1998).
8.   Thomas, D., "The Changing Role of Womanhood: From True Woman to New Woman in Charlotte Perkins Gilman's 'The Yellow Wallpaper,'" http://itech.fgcu.edu/faculty/wohlpart/alra/gilman.htm. See also Gilman, C. P., "Why I Wrote 'The Yellow Wallpaper'?" *The Forerunner*, October 1913, pp. 1920. It is worth noting that, in 1886, when Freud established his practice for treating "nervous diseases," he relied on traditional methods, such as hydrotherapy and the Weir Mitchell rest cure. In 1887, he wrote a favorable review of Mitchell's treatise on the treatment of hysteria. And in 1895, in *Studies in Hysteria*, he wrote: "A combination...between the Breuer and Weir Mitchell procedures produces all the physical improvements that

we expect from the latter, as well as having a far reaching psychical influence such as never results from a rest-cure without psychotherapy." Breuer, J. and Freud, S., *Studies in Hysteria* (1893-1895), *SE.*, vol. 2, pp. xi., 267.

9.   Thomas, D., "The Changing Role of Womanhood," op. cit.
10. Woolf, L., *Beginning Again: An Autobiography of the Years 1911-1918* (New York: Harcourt, Brace & World, 1964), pp. 75-76, 78, emphasis added.
11. Ibid., p. 164.
12. Ibid., p. 79, emphasis added.
13. Ibid., p. 79, emphasis added.
14. Ibid., p. 163.
15. Ibid., p. 256.
16. Spater, G. and Parsons, I., *A Marriage of True Minds: An Intimate Portrait of Leonard and Virginia Woolf* (New York: Harcourt Brace Jovanovich, 1977), p. 69.
17. Woolf, V., "Letter to Violet Dickinson," April 5, 1905. Quoted in Poole, R., *The Unknown Virginia Woolf* (Cambridge: Cambridge University Press, 1978), p. 40.
18. Woolf, V., "Jews," Extracts from Virginia Woolf's 1909 Notebook (Discovered in Birmingham in 2003). http://www.bangla.net/newage/250603/fet.html
19. Woolf, V., "Letter to Madge Vaughan," June 1912. In *Letters*, vol. 1, p. 503.
20. Woolf, V., "Letter to Jacques Raverat," July 30, 1923. Ibid., vol. 3, p. 58, emphasis added.
21. Woolf, V., "Letter to Ethel Smyth," August 2, 1930. Ibid., vol. 4, pp. 195-196.
22. Woolf, V., "Letter to Ethel Smyth," September 28, 1930. Ibid., p. 222.
23. Woolf, V., "Letter to Ethel Smyth," February 28, 1932. Ibid., vol. 5, p. 23.
24. Woolf, V., "Letter to Leonard Woolf," March 18 (?), 1941. Ibid., vol. 6, p. 481.
25. Woolf, V., "Letter to Leonard Woolf," March 28, 1941. Ibid., p. 487.
26. Woolf, L., *Beginning Again*, op. cit., p. 159.
27. Ibid., pp. 178-179.
28. Ibid., p. 80.
29. Szasz, T., *Insanity: The Idea and Its Consequences* [1987] (Syracuse: Syracuse University Press, 1997).
30. Nicolson, N., in Woolf, V., *Letters,* vol. 2, pp. xxxiii-xv.
31. Ibid., p. xiv.
32. Quoted in Coates, I., *Who's Afraid of Leonard Woolf? A Case for the Sanity of Virginia Woolf* (New York: Soho Press, 1998), p. 118.
33. Szasz, T., "On autogenic diseases," *The Freeman*, 54: 24-25 (May), 2004.
34. Zwerdling, A., *Virginia Woolf and the Real World* (Berkeley: University of California Press, 1986), p. 293.
35. Woolf, V., *Diary*, vol. 3, February 16, 1930; quoted in Dunn, J., *A Very Close Conspiracy: Vanessa Bell and Virginia Woolf* (Boston: Little Brown, 1991), pp. 45-46.
36. Zwerdling, A., *Virginia Woolf and the Real World*, op. cit., p. 253.
37. Bell, Q., *Virginia Woolf*, vol. 2, p. 15.
38. Alberoni, F., quoted in Rowland, I. D., "A lesson of September 11," *New York Review of Books*, October 7, 2004, pp. 32-35; p. 35, emphasis added.
39. Poole, R., *The Unknown Virginia Woolf,* op. cit., pp. 250, 251.
40. Woolf, V., *Letters,* vol. 1, p. 488, emphasis added.
41. Ibid., vol, 4, p. 17.
42. Ibid., vol. 4, p. 325, emphasis added.
43. Woolf, V., "Letter to Violet Dickinson," April 11, 1913, *Letters*, vol. 2; quoted in Dunn, J., *A Very Close Conspiracy: Vanessa Bell and Virginia Woolf* (Boston: Little Brown, 1991), p. 190.
44. Woolf, V., *Diary*, September 5, 1926, vol. 3, quoted in Dunn, J., *A Very Close Conspiracy*, op. cit., p. 192.

45.   Woolf, V., *Letters*, vol. 3, 1927; quoted in Dunn, J., *A Very Close Conspiracy*, op. cit., p. 191.

46.   Woolf, V., *Diary*, vol. 1, p. 101, quoted in Zwerdling, A., *Virginia Woolf and the Real World*, op. cit., p. 104.

47.   Zwerdling, A., *Virginia Woolf and the Real World*, op. cit., pp. 233, 98.

48.   Ibid., p. 99.

49.   Woolf, V., *Diary*, vol. 3, p. 230; quoted in Zwerdling, A., *Virginia Woolf and the Real World*, op. cit., pp. 98-99.

50.   It is well to remember in this connection Carl Schmitt's warning about "humanitarianism and universalist international law [as]…particularly glaring instances of liberalism's inconsistent wavering between impotence and immoderation." Muller, J.-W., *A Dangerous Mind: Carl Schmitt and Post-War European Thought* (New Haven, CT: Yale University Press, 2003), p. 33.

Chapter 3. "He shut people up"

1.   Woolf, V., quoted in "ClassicNote on *Mrs. Dalloway*," http://www.gradesaver.com/ClassicNotes/Titles/dalloway/about.html.

2.   Woolf, V., *Mrs. Dalloway* [1925] (New York: Harcourt Brace & World, 1935), p. 134.

3.   Ibid., p. 135.

4.   Ibid., p. 136, emphasis in the original.

5.   Ibid., p. 137.

6.   Ibid., p. 136.

7.   Ibid., pp. 137-138.

8.   Ibid., pp. 150, 153.

9.   Ibid., p. 154.

10.   Freud, S., "A difficulty in the path of psycho-analysis" (1917). *SE*, vol. 17, pp. 135-144; pp. 142, 143.

11.   Poole, R., *The Unknown Virginia Woolf* (Cambridge: Cambridge University Press, 1978), p. 6.

12.   Ibid., p. 1.

13.   Sartre, J-P., *Anti-Semite and Jew* [1948]. Translated by George J. Becker (New York: Schocken Books, 1965), p. 69.

14.   Szasz, T., "Review of *Virginia Woolf: Female Victim of Male Medicine*, by Stephen Trombley," *Inquiry*, December 1982, pp. 44-45.

15.   Poole, R., *The Unknown Virginia Woolf*, op. cit., p. 1.

16.   Ibid., pp. 140-141, emphasis added.

17.   Ibid., p. 189.

18.   Trombley, S., *All That Summer She Was Mad: Virginia Woolf, Female Victim of Male Medicine* (New York: Continuum, 1982), pp. 1, 9.

19.   Ibid., p. 10.

20.   Ibid., p. 5.

21.   Ibid., p. 60.

22.   Bell, Q., *Virginia Woolf*, vol., 2, p. 170.

23.   Trombley, S., *All That Summer She Was Mad*, op. cit., p. 56.

24.   Quoted in ibid., p. 120, emphasis added.

25.   Ibid., p. 171.

26.   Quoted in ibid., pp. 170-171, emphasis added. *Plus ça change, plus c'est la même chose.* But we have made "progress": The American government, aided by the medical-pharmaceutical complex, has enshrined the "universal love of labels" as

"psychiatric science" and made it one of the nation's leading academic and economic growth industries.

27. Szasz, T., *Insanity: The Idea and Its Consequences* [1987] (Syracuse: Syracuse University Press, 1997).
28. Coates, I., *Who's Afraid of Leonard Woolf? A Case for the Sanity of Virginia Woolf* (New York: Soho Press, 1998).
29. Ibid, p. 11, emphasis added. Coates gives no credit to R. D. Laing for this piece of post-Freudian psychobabble.
30. Ibid., p. 142, emphasis added.
31. Ibid., p. 145.
32. Veronal. http://www.ibiblio.org/herbmed/eclectic/ellingwood/veronal.html
33. Coates, I., *Who's Afraid of Leonard Woolf?* op. cit., p. 145, emphasis added.
34. Ibid., p. 187.
35. Quoted in ibid., pp. 190-191.
36. Ibid., p. 153.

Chapter 4. "My madness saved me"

1. Quoted in Trombley, S., *All That Summer She Was Mad: Virginia Woolf, Female Victim of Male Medicine* (New York: Continuum, 1981), p. x.
2. Schreber, D. P., *Memoirs of My Nervous Illness* [1903]. Translated and edited by Macalpine, I. and Hunter, R. A. (London: Dawson, 1955), p. 55, emphasis in the original. In this connection, see further, Lothane, Z., *In Defense of Schreber: Soul Murder and Psychiatry* (Hillsdale, NJ: Analytic Press, 1992).
3. Quoted in Woolf, L., *The Journey Not the Arrival Matters: An Autobiography of the Years 1939-1969* (New York: Harcourt Brace Jovanovich, 1969), p. 93.
4. Woolf., V., *Letters*, vol. 3, pp. 92-93.
5. Woolf, V., *A Writer's Diary: Being Extracts from the Diary of Virginia Woolf*, edited by Leonard Woolf (New York: Signet/New American Library, 1968), p. 197.
6. See Stone, M., "Life-Lies and Self-Deceptions," http://www.thephaneronpress.com/publications.html. Peterson, J. B., "The Pragmatics of Meaning," http://www.semioticon.com/frontline/jordan_b.htm.
7. Woolf, V., *A Room of One's Own* [1929] (New York: Harvest Books, 1989), p. 115.
8. Woolf., V., *Letters*, vol. 4, p. 180.
9. See Szasz, T., *Insanity: The Idea and Its Consequences* [1987] (Syracuse: Syracuse University Press, 1997).
10. Meisel, P. and Kendrick, W., editors. *Bloomsbury/Freud: The Letters of James and Alix Strachey, 1925-1925* (New York: Basic Books, 1985), p. 190.
11. Ibid., p. 198.
12. Ibid., p. 211, emphasis in the original.
13. Szasz, T., "The secular cure of souls: 'Analysis' or dialogue?" *Existential Analysis*, 14: 203-212 (July), 2003.
14. Greenberg, J. (Hannah Green), *I Never Promised You a Rose Garden* (New York: Holt, Rinehart & Winston, 1964).
15. Greenberg, J., "Self-deceit is a strong fort," in Stern, C., editor, *Gates of Repentance: The New Union Prayer Book for the Days of Awe* (New York: Central Conference of American Rabbis), 1978, p. 237. Quoted in Silver, A. S., "Frieda Fromm-Reichmann, loneliness, and deafness," *International Forum of Psychoanalysis,* 5: 39-46, 1996, p. 39.
16. Bell, Q., *Virginia Woolf*, vol. 2, pp. 19, 20.
17. Woolf, L., *Downhill All the Way: An Autobiography of the Years 1919-1939* (New York: Vintage, 1967), p. 164.

18.   Woolf, V., *Diary*, vol. 1, p. 110.
19.   Ibid., p. 221, emphasis added.
20.   Woolf, V., *Letters*, vol. 2, p. 369.
21.   Ibid., p. 482.
22.   Woolf, V., *Diary*, vol. 2, p. 242.
23.   Woolf, V., *Letters*, vol. 3, p. 43.
24.   Woolf, V., *Diary*, vol. 1, p. p. 302. The abbreviation "P.S.S." has remained undeciphered.
25.   Woolf, V., *Letters*, vol. 3, p. 132.
26.   Ibid., p. 133.
27.   Ibid., pp. 134-135.
28.   Ibid., vol. 5, p. 36.
29.   Woolf, V., *Diary*, vol. 2, p. 322.
30.   Woolf, V., *Letters*, vol. 3, p. 381.
31.   Ibid., vol. 5, p. 37.
32.   Quoted in, Clark, R. W., *Freud: The Man and The Cause* (London: Jonathan Cape & Weidenfeld & Nicolson, 1980), p. 417.
33.   Szasz, T., *The Myth of Psychotherapy: Mental Healing as Religion, Rhetoric, and Repression* [1978] (Syracuse: Syracuse University Press, 1988).
34.   Quoted in Roazen, P., *Freud and His Followers* (New York: Knopf, 1975), p. 347, emphasis added.
35.   Bond, A. H., *Who Killed Virginia Woolf? A Psychobiography* (New York: Human Sciences Press, 1989), p. 11.
36.   Abel, E., *Virginia Woolf and the Fictions of Psychoanalysis* (Chicago: University of Chicago Press, 1989), pp. xvi, xvii, emphasis added.
37.   Ibid., p. xvi.
38.   See Hyman, S. E., *The Tangled Bank: Darwin, Marx, Frazer, and Freud as Imaginative Writers* (New York: Athenaeum, 1962); Szasz, T., *Anti-Freud: Karl Kraus's Criticism of Psychoanalysis and Psychiatry* [1976] (Syracuse: Syracuse University Press, 1990).
39.   Jouve, N. W., "Virginia Woolf and psychoanalysis," in Roe, S. and Sellers, S., editors, *The Cambridge Companion to Virginia Woolf* (Cambridge: Cambridge University Press, 2000), pp. 245-272.
40.   Ibid., p. 245.
41.   Ibid.
42.   Ibid., p. 247.
43.   Ibid., p. 246.
44.   http://www.psychoanalysis.org.uk/archivesexhibition.htm
45.   Freud, S., "History of the Psycho-Analytic Movement" (1914), *SE*, vol. 14, p. 7.
46.   Freud, S., *An Outline of Psychoanalysis* (1940), *SE*, vol. 23, p. 197. Freud compares psychoanalysis with the microscope.
47.   Freud, S., *The Question of Lay Analysis* (1927), *SE*, vol. 20, p. 187.
48.   Szasz, T., *The Meaning of Mind: Language, Morality, and Neuroscience* [1996] (Syracuse: Syracuse University Press, 2002).
49.   Szasz, T., *The Ethics of Psychoanalysis: The Theory and Method of Autonomous Psychotherapy* [1965] (Syracuse: Syracuse University Press, 1988).
50.   Freud, S., "History of the Psycho-Analytic Movement" (1914), *SE*, vol. 14, p. 49.
51.   Ibid., p. 49.
52.   Freud, S., *An Outline of Psychoanalysis* (1940), *SE*, vol. 23, p. 174.
53.   Freud, S., "History of the Psycho-Analytic Movement" (1914), *SE*, vol. 14, p. 64.
54.   Hyman, S. E., *The Tangled Bank: Darwin, Marx, Frazer, and Freud as Imaginative Writers* (New York: Athenaeum, 1962), p. 313.

55. Freud, S., "Psychoanalysis and the establishment of the facts in legal proceedings" (1906), *SE*, vol. 9, pp. 97-114; p. 108.

56. Freud, S., *New Introductory Lectures* (1932), *SE*, vol. 22, p. 155, emphasis added.

57. Woolf, V., *A Room of One's Own* [1929] (New York: Harvest Books, 1989), pp. 50-51.

58. Clark, R. W., *Freud*, op. cit., p. 422.

59. Meng, M., "Freud and the sculptor" (1956), in Ruitenbeek, H. M., editor, *Freud As We Knew Him* (Detroit: Wayne State University Press, 1973), pp. 350-352; p. 351.

Chapter 5. "A screwed up shrunk very old man"

1. Freud, S., "Preface to Marie Bonaparte's *The Life and Works of Edgar Allan Poe: A Psycho-Analytic Interpretation*" (1933), *SE*, vol. 22, p. 254.

2. Zweig, S., "Portrait of Freud" (1932), in Ruitenbeek, H. M., editor, *Freud As We Knew Him* (Detroit: Wayne State University Press, 1973), pp. 90-97; p. 93. Excerpt from Zweig, S., *Mental Healers: Franz Anton Mesmer, Mary Baker Eddy, Sigmund Freud* [1932], translated by Eden and Cedar Paul (New York: Frederick Ungar, 1962).

3. Quoted in Clark, R. W., *Freud: The Man and The Cause* (London: Jonathan Cape & Weidenfeld & Nicolson, 1980), p. 418, emphasis added.

4. Quoted in Lehman, H., "Sigmund Freud and Thomas Mann," (1970), in Ruitenbeek, H. M., editor, *Freud As We Knew Him*, op. cit., pp. 504-517; p. 511.

5. Freud, S., "The Moses of Michelangelo" (1914), *SE*, vol. 13, pp. 209-238; p. 211.

6. Ibid.

7. Ibid., p. 212, emphasis added.

8. Ibid., emphasis added.

9. Ibid., emphasis added

10. Freud, S., "Preface to Marie Bonaparte's *The Life and Works of Edgar Allan Poe* ," op. cit., p. 254.

11. Freud, S., "The Moses of Michelangelo," op. cit., p. 212; and "Leonardo da Vinci and a memory of his childhood" (1910), *SE*, vol. 11, pp. 57-137; p. 63.

12. Freud, S. and Bullitt, W. C. *Thomas Woodrow Wilson, Twenty-eighth President of the United States: A Psychological Study* (Boston: Houghton Mifflin, 1967). See also Szasz, T., *Karl Kraus and the Soul-Doctors: A Pioneer Critic and His Criticism of Psychiatry and Psychoanalysis* (Baton Rouge: Louisiana State University Press, 1976); reprinted, *Anti-Freud: Karl Kraus's Criticism of Psychoanalysis and Psychiatry* (Syracuse: Syracuse University Press, 1990).

13. Freud, S., "Leonardo da Vinci and a memory of his childhood," op. cit., p. 63.

14. Ibid., p. 68.

15. Ibid., p. 69.

16. Ibid., pp. 71-72.

17. This is based on a childhood memory, or possibly dream, of Leonardo's in which he claimed that, as an infant, a kite flew down, opened his [Leonardo's] lips with its tail feathers, and with its tail struck his lips several times.

18 . Freud, S., "Leonardo da Vinci and a memory of his childhood," op. cit., p. 85.

19. Ibid., p. 87.

20. Freud, S., "The Moses of Michelangelo," op. cit., p. 212, emphasis added.

21. Freud, S. and Bullitt, W. C., *Thomas Woodrow Wilson, Twenty-eighth President of the United States*, op. cit.

22. Marcuse, L., "Freud's Aesthetics" (1958), in Ruitenbeek, H. M., editor, *Freud As We Knew Him*, op. cit., pp. 385-411; p. 395.

23. Zweig, S., "Portrait of Freud," op. cit., p. 94.
24. Laforgue, R., "Personal Memories of Freud" (1956), in Ruitenbeek, H. M., editor, *Freud As We Knew Him*, op. cit., pp. 341-349; p. 348.
25. Clark, R. W., *Freud*, op. cit., p. 467.
26. Papini, G., http://translate.google.com/translate?hl=en&sl=it&u=http://www.volontari.org/papini.html&prev=search%3Fq%3Dgiovanni%2Bpapini%26hl%3Den%26lr%3D%26ie%3DUTF8%26sa%3DG; and http://www.kirjasto.sci.fi/papini.htm.
27. See "Review, *Picasso: The Communist Years*, by Gertje R. Utley," http://www.101investing.com/products/ASIN0300082517.php.
28. My summary of Papini's imagined visit with Freud is based on Papini, G., "A Visit to Freud" (1934), in Ruitenbeek, H. M., editor, *Freud As We Knew Him*, op. cit., pp. 98-102. Although the interview was fictitious, Ruitenbeek did not know it and presented it as genuine. See Crews, F. C., "In response to *The Unknown Freud*" (Letters), *New York Review of Books*, 40: 56 (December 16, 1993).
29. Papini, G., "A Visit to Freud," op. cit., p. 99.
30. Ibid., p. 100.
31. Ibid.
32. Ibid., emphasis added.
33. Ibid., p. 101.
34. Ibid., pp. 101-102.
35. Bell, Q., *Virginia Woolf*, vol. 2, p. 209.

Chapter 6. "He will go on, better without me"

1. Stephen, L., *The Science of Ethics* (London: Smith Eder, 1882), pp. 391-392.
2. Woolf, L., *The Journey Not the Arrival Matters: An Autobiography of the Years 1939-1969* (New York: Harcourt Brace Jovanovich, 1969), p. 15.
3. Ibid., pp. 11, 16.
4. Ibid., p. 73.
5. Ibid.
6. Ibid., p. 46.
7. Quoted in Ingram, I. M., "Virginia Woolf's psychiatric history," http://ourworld.compuserve.com/homepages/malcolmi/suicide.htm. Subsequent quotations are from this source, unless otherwise identified.
8. Ibid.
9. Ibid.
10. Woolf, V., *Mrs. Dalloway* [1925] (New York: Harcourt Brace & World, 1935), p. 136, emphasis in the original.
11. Ingram, I. M., "Virginia Woolf's psychiatric history," op. cit.
12. Woolf, L., *The Journey Not the Arrival Matters*, op. cit., pp. 90-91.
13. Ibid., pp. 93-94, emphasis added.
14. Ibid., p. 93.
15. Ibid., pp. 93-94.
16. Poole, R., *The Unknown Virginia Woolf* (Cambridge: Cambridge University Press, 1978), p. 169.
17. Bond, A. H., *Who Killed Virginia Woolf? A Psychobiography* (New York: Human Sciences Press, 1989), p. 160.
18. Woolf, L., *The Journey Not the Arrival Matters*, op. cit., p. 91.
19. Ibid., emphasis added.
20. Ibid., emphasis added.

21. Ibid., pp. 91-92.
22. Ibid., pp. 92-93.
23. Bell, Q., *Virginia Woolf*, vol. 2, p. 224, emphasis added.
24. Ingram, I. M., "Virginia Woolf's psychiatric history," op. cit.
25. Karin Stephen, who too was said to be suffering from manic-depression, also committed suicide. See Rossdale, P. and Robinson, K., "Bloomsbury and Psychoanalysis: An Exhibition of Documents from the Archives of the British Psychoanalytical Society," http://www.psychoanalysis.org.uk/archivesexhibition.htm.
26. Szasz, T., *Fatal Freedom: The Ethics and Politics of Suicide* [1999] (Syracuse: Syracuse University Press, 2002).
27. Szasz, T., *Sex By Prescription: The Startling Truth About Today's Sex Therapy* [1980] (Syracuse: Syracuse University Press, 1990).
28. Aquinas, St. Thomas, *Summa Theologica*, IIII, 154, 11. http://www.fordham.edu/halsall/source/aquinashomo.html
29. "Sex: Natural vs Unnatural, Categorizing Unnatural Sex," http://www.trosch.org/the/sex_nvun.html#unnatural.
30. Szasz, T., *The Manufacture of Madness: A Comparative Study of the Inquisition and the Mental Health Movement* [1970] (Syracuse: Syracuse University Press, 1997).
31. Magrane, B. P., Gilliland, M. G. F., and King, D. E., "Certification of death by family physicians," http://www.aafp.org/afp/971001ap/magrane.html.
32. Goethe, J. W., *Dichtung und Wahrheit (Poetry and Truth)*, in Goethe, J. W., *Gedenkausgabe der Werke, Briefe und Gespräche* (24 vols.; Zurich und Stuttgart: Artemis Verlag, 1962), p. 637; Goethe, J. W., *Autobiography*, in Goethe, J. W., *The Complete Works of Johann Wolfgang von Goethe*, translated by John Oxenford (10 vols.; New York: P. F. Collier & Son, n.d.), vol. 2, p. 163. Freely translated by me. John Oxenford offers this translation: "Suicide is an event of human nature, which, whatever may be said and done with respect to it, demands the sympathy of every man, and in every epoch must be discussed anew."

Chapter 7. "He's got a finger in my mind"

1. "Books and Writers. Virginia Woolf (1882-1941)," http://www.readprint.com/author-91/Virginia-Woolf.
2. Woolf, V., "Letter to Ethel Smyth," January 12, 1941, *Letters*, vol. 4, p. 333.
3. Glendinning, V., *Vita: The Life of V. Sackville-West* (London: Weidenfeld & Nicolson, 1983), pp. 139-140.
4. Ibid., p. 149.
5. Ibid., pp. 150-151.
6. Woolf, V., *Letters*, vol. 4, p. 333, emphasis added.
7. Woolf, V., *Mrs. Dalloway* [1925] (New York: Harcourt Brace & World, 1935), p. 281, emphasis added.
8. Woolf, V., *Letters*, vol. 3, p. 381.
9. Ibid., p. 155.
10. Woolf, V., *On Being Ill* (London: Hogarth Press, 1930), p. 22.
11. Ibid., p. 18.

Appendix I. Virginia Woolf, Mad Genius

1. See Szasz, T., *The Meaning of Mind: Language, Morality, and Neuroscience* [1996] (Syracuse: Syracuse University Press, 2002); Jacobs, J., *Choosing Character: Responsibility for Virtue and Vice* (Ithaca, NY: Cornell University Press, 2001).

2. Heschel, A. J., *The Prophets* (New York: Harper & Row, 1962), p. 392.
3. "German Epilepsy Museum Kork," http://www.epilepsie museum.de/alt/body_prominenteen.html; "Famous people with epilepsy," http://www.epilepsy.com/epilepsy/famous.html. See also http://yourmedicalsource.com/library/epilepsy/EPI_whatis.html.
4. "The History of Human Tuberculosis," www.wits.ac.za/myco/html/h_tb.htm-22k; "Famous People Diagnosed With Tuberculosis," http://www.state.de.us/dhss/dph/dpc/tbfamouspeople.html; "List of famous tuberculosis victims," http://www.brainyencyclopedia.com/encyclopedia/l/li/list_of_famous_tuberculosis_victims.html.
5. "A scientist, a patriot, a genius," *U.S. News & World Report,* November 5, 2001, p. 12.
6. Diamond, E. A., "Kay R. Jamison, Ph.D., gives personal perspective on manic depressive illness," *Psychiatric Times,* vol. 18, Issue 7, July 2001. http://www.psychiatrictimes.com/p010701a.html. Compare Jamison's confidence that human behavior, even one as complexly motivated as "manic-depression," is genetically determined, with the reservations of distinguished geneticists: "For the truth is, of course, that we have little idea how much of the variation in human behavior…is caused by genes." H. Allen Orr, "Vive la difference!" *New York Review of Books*, May 12, 2005, pp. 19-20; p. 20. "It is remarkable how little we really know about the genetics of human behaviour." Coyne, J. A., "Legends of Linnaeus: When 'Europeans were governed by laws, Asians by opinions and Africans by caprice,'" *TLS*, February 25, 2005, pp. 3-4; p. 3.
7. King, J., *Virginia Woolf* (New York: Norton, 1994), p. xviii.
8. Jamison, K. R., "Afterword," in Caramagno, T. C., *The Flight of the Mind: Virginia Woolf's Art and Manic-Depressive Illness*, with an Afterword by Kay Redfield Jamison (Berkeley: University of California Press, 1992), pp. 303-305; p. 303.
9. Jamison, K. R., "Kay Jamison touches the fire," http://www.wga.org/health/jamison/touchedfull.html, emphasis added.
10. Jamison, K. R., "Afterword," in Caramagno, T. C., *The Flight of the Mind*, op. cit., p. 303.
11. Jamison, K. R., "Kay Jamison touches the fire," op. cit., emphasis added.
12. Jamison, K. R., "Afterword," in Caramagno, T. C., *The Flight of the Mind*, op. cit., p. 304, emphasis added; Goodwin, F. K. and Jamison, K. R., *Manic-Depressive Illness* (New York: Oxford University Press, 1990), p. 3.
13. Quoted in Butterfield, F., "Massachusetts Gun Laws Concerning Mentally Ill Are Faulted," *New York Times*, January 14, 2001, Internet edition.
14. Jamison, K. R., *An Unquiet Mind: A Memoir of Mood and Madness* (New York: Knopf, 1995), p. 113.
15. "Lithium Lessons Learned," *Psychiatric News*, 38: 27 (April 18), 2003. http://pn.psychiatryonline.org/cgi/content/full/38/8/27?etoc
16. Masur, K. and Chang, S., "Interview with Dr. Kay Redfield Jamison," March 3, 1998. http://www.livefromlincolncenter.org/backstage/march3/jamison.htm, emphasis added.
17. Gutin, J.A.C., "The science of creativity: That fine madness—manic depression is latest mental illness popularly linked to artistic genius," *Discover*, October 1996. http://www.findarticles.com/p/articles/mi_m1511/is_n10_v17/ai_18693671
18. Jamison, K. R., *Exuberance: The Passion for Life* (New York: Knopf, 2004); Simon, C. C., "Exuberance: Four cheers for this little-understood, often mocked, slightly scary emotion," *Washington Post*, September 28, 2004, p. H1. http://www.washingtonpost.com/wpdyn/articles/A552282004Sep27.html

19. Simon, C. C., "Exuberance: Four cheers for this little-understood, often mocked, slightly scary emotion," op. cit., emphasis added.

20. Szasz, T., *Fatal Freedom: The Ethics and Politics of Suicide* [1999] (Syracuse: Syracuse University Press, 2002), pp. 54-58.

21. Goodwin, F. K. and Jamison, K. R., *Manic-Depressive Illness*, op. cit., p. 774.

22. Ibid., emphasis added.

23. Ibid., p. 782.

24. Jamison, K. R., *Touched With Fire: Manic Depressive Illness and the Artistic Temperament* (New York: The Free Press, 1993), p. 250.

25. Artaud, A., "Van Gogh, the Man Suicided by Society" [1947], in Artaud, A., *Selected Writings*, edited by Susan Sontag, translated by Helen Weaver (New York: Farrar, Straus and Giroux, 1976), pp. 496-497.

26. Jamison, K. R., *Touched With Fire*, op. cit., p. 239. Jamison imitates Francis Galton's "method" set forth in his famous book, *Hereditary Genius* (1869), where "he assembled long lists of 'eminent' men—judges, poets, scientists, even oarsmen and wrestlers—to show that excellence ran in families." Holt, J., "Measure for measure: The strange science of Francis Galton," *New Yorker*, January 24 & 31, 2005, pp. 84-90; p. 85.

27. Martinetti, R., "Hemingway: A Look Back," *American Authors*, http://www.americanlegends.com/authors/.

28. Jamison, K. R., *Touched With Fire*, op. cit., p. 228.

29. Hotchner, A. E., *Papa Hemingway: A Personal Memoir* [1966] (New York: Bantam Books, 1967), p. 304.

30. Ibid., p. 308.

31. Ibid., p. 321.

32. Ibid., p. 324.

33. Ibid.

34. Ibid., pp. 328, 330.

35. Ibid., 331.

36. Caramagno, T. C., *The Flight of the Mind*, op. cit., p. 1. Cited from "Bipolar Disorder & Virginia Woolf," http://www.caramagnobooks.com/77724.html.

37. For a critique, see Szasz, T., *Pharmacracy: Medicine and Politics in America* [2001] (Syracuse: Syracuse University Press, 2003).

38. "Bipolar Disorder & Virginia Woolf," http://www.caramagnobooks.com/77724.html, emphasis added.

39. Ibid.

40. Ibid., emphasis added.

41. Caramagno, T. C., *The Flight of the Mind*, op. cit., p. 296.

42. Flaherty, A. W., *The Midnight Disease: The Drive to Write, Writer's Block, and the Creative Brain* (Boston: Houghton Mifflin Company, 2004), dust jacket.

43. Szasz, T., *A Lexicon of Lunacy: Metaphoric Malady, Moral Responsibility, and Psychiatry* (New Brunswick, NJ: Transaction Publishers, 1993).

44. Flaherty, A. W., *The Midnight Disease*, op. cit., p. 7.

45. See Szasz, T., *Pharmacracy*, op. cit.

46. Flaherty, A. W., *The Midnight Disease*, op. cit., p. 8, emphasis added.

47. Ibid., pp. 34, 35, emphasis added.

48. Ibid., p. 234.

49. Szegedy-Maszak, M., "Wired by words," http://www.usnews.com/usnews/issue/040216/health/16conv.htm.

50. Ibid., emphasis added.

51. Dupree, C., "Muse of the hemispheres: Authorial synapses," *Harvard Magazine*, JanuaryFebruary 2004. http://www.harvardmagazine.com/online/010441.html, emphasis added.
52. Ibid., emphasis added.
53. Ussher, J. M., *Women's Madness: Misogyny or Mental Illness?* (Amherst: University of Massachusetts Press, 1991), p. 3, emphasis added.
54. Ibid., p. 4.
55. Ibid., p. 5.
56. Ibid.
57. Ibid., p. 11.
58. Ibid., p. 220.
59. South Australian Consolidated Acts, Mental Health Act 1993. http://www.austlii.edu.au/au/legis/sa/consol_act/mha1993128/s12.html
60. Ussher, J. M., *Women's Madness*, op. cit., p. 220.
61. I explain what I mean when I say that such relationships are "prohibited" in *Liberation By Oppression: A Comparative Study of Slavery and Psychiatry* (New Brunswick, NJ: Transaction, 2002), especially pp. 35-54.
62. Szasz, T., *Pharmacracy,* op. cit.
63. Ussher, J. M., *Women's Madness*, op. cit., p. 221, emphasis added.
64. Ibid., p. 55.
65. Ibid., p. 254.
66. Ibid., p. 306.
67. The contemporary expert on human behavior and mental illness is mesmerized by the image of people "being driven crazy"—by alcohol, illegal drugs, gambling, jealousy, money, war, work, and, of course, "trauma." Columnist Charles Krauthammer (an ex-psychiatrist) joins the chorus proclaiming a "proximity between genius and madness," which, in the case of chess at least, he attributes to the game, not to genes. Characterizing former world champion chess player Bobby Fischer as "clearly a sick man...the poster boy for the mad chess genius," Krauthammer ridicules his "insane rants about Jews" and "paranoia," and belittles him by comparing him to Natan Sharansky, "the sanest man I know [and] a chess master who once played Gary Kasparov to a draw." Krauthammer, C., "Did chess make him crazy?" *Time*, May 2, 2005, p. 96.

Appendix II. The Mad Genius Problem

1. Anthony Storr, "The darkness that has brought us light," *The Weekend Review/The Independent* (London), March 20, 1999, p. 11.
2. Szasz, T., *Insanity: The Idea and Its Consequences* (New York: Wiley, 1987); with a new Preface (Syracuse: Syracuse University Press, 1990).
3. Becker, G., *The Mad Genius Controversy: A Study in the Sociology of Deviance* (Beverly Hills, CA: Sage Publications, 1978), p. 25.
4. Ibid., p. 24.
5. Ibid., pp. 29, 30.
6. For example, See Gleick, J., *Genius: The Life and Science of Richard Feynman* (New York: Pantheon, 1992), and Joan Acocella's long Preface in Nijinsky, V., *The Diary of Vaslav Nijinsky*. (Unexpurgated Edition), translated by Kyril Fitzlyon, edited by Joan Acocella (New York: Farrar, Straus and Giroux, 1995).
7. Pickover, C. A., *Strange Brains and Genius: The Secret Lives of Eccentric Scientists and Madmen* (New York: Plenum, 1998).
8. Gleick, J., op. cit. Quoted from http://www.cc.gatech.edu/people/home/idris/Essays/Gleick_Genius_Excerpt.htm.

9. The John D. and Catherine T. MacArthur Foundation has no trouble finding 20-30 persons—who must be residents or citizens of the United States—every year deserving of its "Genius Award" ("Fellowship").
10. Kretschmer, E., *The Psychology of Men of Genius* [1931]. Translated and with an introduction by R. B. Cattell (College Park, MD: McGrath Publishing Company, 1970). Kretschmer states that the book was originally written in 1919.
11. Holt, J., "Measure for measure: The strange science of Francis Galton," *New Yorker*, January 24 and 31, 2005, pp. 84-90; p. 85. http://www.newyorker.com/critics/books/?050124crbo_books.
12. See Appendix I.
13. Holt, J., "Measure for measure," op. cit.
14. Trofim Denisovich Lysenko (1898-1976) was an agronomist and the "inventor" of a new agricultural technique, vernalization, that promised to triple or quadruple agricultural yields. See "Lysenkoism," http://en.wikipedia.org/wiki/Lysenkoism.
15. The image of a "superior race" is the eugenic-scientist version of the religious image of a "chosen people."
16. Lombroso, C., quoted at http://www.bellaonline.com/articles/art15908.asp.
17. Carra, G. and Barale, F., "Images in Psychiatry: Cesare Lombroso, M.D., 1835–1909," *American Journal of Psychiatry*, 161: 624-625 (April) 2004. http://ajp.psychiatryonline.org/cgi/content/full/161/4/624. Lombroso was Jewish.
18. Kretschmer, E., *The Psychology of Men of Genius*, op. cit., p. 14.
19. Ibid., pp. 6, 12.
20. Cattell, R. B., "Translator's Foreword," in ibid., pp. vii-x; p. vii, emphasis added.
21. Ibid., p. ix.
22. Ibid.
23. "Edward Munch's Biography," http://www.worldartsales.net/sample/munch.htm.
24. "Web Museum: Rubens, Peter Paul," http://www.ibiblio.org/wm/paint/auth/rubens/.
25. Schjeldahl, P., "Rubenessence," *New Yorker*, February 7, 2005, pp. 88-89; p. 89, emphasis added.
26. BBC Radio 4: "Relatively Einstein," http://www.bbc.co.uk/radio4/science/relativelyeinstein.shtml.

Bibliography

Abel, E., *Virginia Woolf and the Fictions of Psychoanalysis* (Chicago: University of Chicago Press, 1989).

Artaud, A., *Selected Writings*. Edited by Susan Sontag. Translated by Helen Weaver (New York: Farrar, Straus and Giroux, 1976).

Auden, W. H., *The Dyer's Hand, and Other Essays* [1962] (New York: Vintage, 1968).

Baker, C., *Ernest Hemingway: A Life Story* [1968] (New York: Bantam Books, 1970).

Becker, G., *The Mad Genius Controversy: A Study in the Sociology of Deviance* (Beverly Hills, CA: Sage Publications, 1978).

Bell, Q., *Virginia Woolf: A Biography* (2 vols.; New York: Harcourt Brace Jovanovich, 1972).

Bond, A. H., *Who Killed Virginia Woolf? A Psychobiography* (New York: Human Sciences Press, 1989).

Bredvold, L. T. and Ross, R. G., editors, *The Philosophy of Edmund Burke, A Selection from his Speeches and Writings* (Ann Arbor, MI: University of Michigan Press, 1960).

Caplan, A. L., McCartney, J. J., and Sisti, D. A., editors, *Health, Disease, and Illness: Concepts in Medicine* (Washington, D.C.: Georgetown University Press, 2004).

Caramagno, T. C., *The Flight of the Mind: Virginia Woolf's Art and Manic-Depressive Illness*. With an Afterword by Kay Redfield Jamison (Berkeley: University of California Press, 1992).

Clark, R. W., *Freud: The Man and The Cause* (London: Jonathan Cape & Weidenfeld & Nicolson, 1980).

Coates, I., *Who's Afraid of Leonard Woolf? A Case for the Sanity of Virginia Woolf* (New York: Soho Press, 1998).

DeSalvo, L., *Conceived with Malice: Literature as Revenge in the Lives and Works of Virginia and Leonard Woolf, D. H. Lawrence, Djuna Barnes, and Henry Miller* (New York: Dutton, 1994).

DeSalvo, L., *Virginia Woolf: The Impact of Childhood Sexual Abuse on her Life and Work* (New York: Ballantine Books, 1989).

DeSalvo, L., *Writing as a Way of Healing: How Telling Our Stories Transforms Our Lives* (San Francisco: Harper, 1999).

Diller, J. V., *Freud's Jewish Identity: A Case Study in the Impact of Ethnicity* (Rutherford, N.J.: Farleigh Dickinson University Press, 1991).

Dunn, J., *A Very Close Conspiracy: Vanessa Bell and Virginia Woolf* (Boston: Little Brown, 1991).

Flaherty, A. W., *The Midnight Disease: The Drive to Write, Writer's Block, and the Creative Brain* (Boston: Houghton, Mifflin, 2004).

Freud, S., *The Standard Edition of the Complete Psychological Works of Sigmund Freud.* Translated by James Strachey (24 vols.; London: Hogarth Press, 1953-1974).

Freud, S. and Bullitt, W. C. *Thomas Woodrow Wilson, Twenty-eighth President of the United States: A Psychological Study* (Boston: Houghton Mifflin, 1967).

Galton, F., *Hereditary Genius: An Inquiry into Its Laws and Consequences* [1869] (Magnolia, MA: Peter Smith, 1990).

Gilman, C. P., *The Yellow Wallpaper* [1892]. Edited by Dale M. Bauer (Boston: Belford/St. Martin's, 1998).

Gleick, J., *Genius: The Life and Science of Richard Feynman* (New York: Pantheon, 1992).

Glendinning, V., *Vita: The Life of V. Sackville-West* (London: Weidenfeld & Nicolson, 1983).

Glenny, A., *Ravenous Identity: Eating and Eating Distress in the Life and Work of Virginia Woolf* (New York: St. Martin's Press, 1999).

Goethe, J. W., *The Complete Works of Johann Wolfgang von Goethe.* Translated by John Oxenford (10 vols.; New York: P. F. Collier & Son, n.d.).

Goethe, J. W., *Gedenkausgabe der Werke, Briefe und Gespräche* (24 vols.; Zurich und Stuttgart: Artemis Verlag, 1962).

Goffman, E., *Asylums: Essays on the Social Situation of Mental Patients and Other Inmates* (Garden City, N.Y.: Doubleday Anchor, 1961).

Goodwin, F. K. and Jamison, K. R., *Manic-Depressive Illness* (New York: Oxford University Press, 1990).

Heschel, A. J., *The Prophets* (New York: Harper & Row, 1962).

Hotchner, A. E., *Papa Hemingway: A Personal Memoir* [1966] (New York: Bantam Books, 1967).

Hubert, S. J., *Questions of Power: The Politics of Women's Madness Narratives* (Honolulu: University of Hawaii Press, 2003).

Hyman, S. E., *The Tangled Bank: Darwin, Marx, Frazer and Freud as Imaginative Writers* (New York: Atheneum, 1962).

Hyslop, T. B., *The Great Abnormals* (London: Philip Allan & Co., 1925).

Jacobs, J., *Choosing Character: Responsibility for Virtue and Vice* (Ithaca, N.Y.: Cornell University Press, 2001).

Janeway, E., *Powers of the Weak* (New York: Knopf, 1980).

Jamison, K. R., *Exuberance: The Passion for Life* (New York: Knopf, 2004).

Jamison, K. R., *Night Falls Fast: Understanding Suicide* (New York: Knopf, 1999).

Jamison, K. R., *Touched With Fire: Manic-Depressive Illness and the Artistic Temperament* (New York: The Free Press, 1993).

Jamison, K. R., *An Unquiet Mind: A Memoir of Mood* and *Madness* (New York: Knopf, 1995).

Jones, E., *The Life and Work of Sigmund Freud* (3 vols.; New York: Basic Books, 1953-1957).

King, J., *Virginia Woolf* (New York: Norton, 1994).

Kretschmer, E., *The Psychology of Men of Genius* [1931]. Translated and with an introduction by R. B. Cattell (College Park, MD: McGrath Publishing Company, 1970).

Lee, H., *Virginia Woolf* (New York: A. A. Knopf, 1997).

Lehman, J., *Thrown to the Woolfs* (London: Weidenfeld and Nicolson, 1978).

Lothane, Z., *In Defense of Schreber: Soul Murder and Psychiatry* (Hillsdale, N.J.: Analytic Press, 1992).

Lytton, R. B., *A Blighted Life: A True Story* [1880] (Bristol, U.K.: Thoemmes Press, 1994).

Maze, J., *Virginia Woolf: Feminism, Creativity, and the Unconscious* (Westpost, CT: Greenwood Press, 1997).

Meisel, P. and Kendrick, W., editors, *Bloomsbury/Freud: The Letters of James and Alix Strachey, 1924-1925* (New York: Basic Books, 1985).

Mitchell, L., *Bulwer Lytton: The Rise and Fall of a Victorian Man of Letters* (London: Hambledon & London, 2003).

Moore, G. E., *Principia Ethica* [1903] (Cambridge: Cambridge University Press, 1956).

Morizot, C. A., *Just This Side of Madness: Creativity and the Drive to Create* (Houston, TX: Harold House, 1978).

Muller, J.-W., *A Dangerous Mind: Carl Schmitt and Post-War European Thought* (New Haven, CT: Yale University Press, 2003).

Nijinsky, V., *The Diary of Vaslav Nijinsky*. (Unexpurgated Edition.) Translated by Kyril Fitzlyon, edited by Joan Acocella (New York: Farrar, Straus and Giroux, 1995).

Nunez, S., *Mitz: The Marmoset of Bloomsbury* (New York: HarperFlamingo, 1998).

Pickover, C. A., *Strange Brains and Genius: The Secret Lives Of Eccentric Scientists and Madmen* (New York: Plenum, 1998).

Poole, R., *The Unknown Virginia Woolf* (Cambridge: Cambridge University Press, 1978).

Roazen, P., *Freud and His Followers* (New York: Knopf, 1975).

Roe, S. and Sellers, S., editors, *The Cambridge Companion to Virginia Woolf* (Cambridge: Cambridge University Press, 2000).

Rosenfeld, N., *Outsiders Together: Virginia and Leonard Woolf* (Princeton: Princeton University Press, 2000).

Ruitenbeek, H. M., editor, *Freud As We Knew Him* (Detroit: Wayne State University Press, 1973).

Russell, B., *Unpopular Essays* (New York: Simon and Schuster, 1950).

Sartre, J-P., *Anti-Semite and Jew* [1948]. Translated by George J. Becker (New York: Schocken Books, 1965).

Schreber, D. P., *Memoirs of My Nervous Illness* [1903]. Translated and edited by Macalpine, I. and Hunter, R. A. (London: Dawson, 1955).

Skidelsky, R., *John Maynard Keynes: Volume One, Hopes Betrayed, 1883-1920* (New York: Viking, 1986).

Spater, G. and Parsons, I., *A Marriage of True Minds: An Intimate Portrait of Leonard and Virginia Woolf* (New York: Harcourt Brace Jovanovich, 1977).

Stephen, L., *The Science of Ethics* (London: Smith Eder, 1882).

Szasz, T., *Anti-Freud: Karl Kraus's Criticism of Psychoanalysis and Psychiatry* [1976] (Syracuse: Syracuse University Press, 1990).

Szasz, T., *Ceremonial Chemistry: The Ritual Persecution of Drugs, Addicts, and Pushers* [1976] (Syracuse: Syracuse University Press, 2003).

Szasz, T., *Cruel Compassion: The Psychiatric Control of Society's Unwanted* [1994] (Syracuse: Syracuse University Press, 1998).

Szasz, T., *The Ethics of Psychoanalysis: The Theory and Method of Autonomous Psychotherapy* [1965] (Syracuse: Syracuse University Press, 1988).

Szasz, T., *Fatal Freedom: The Ethics and Politics of Suicide* [1999] (Syracuse: Syracuse University Press, 2002).

Szasz, T., *Ideology and Insanity: Essays on the Psychiatric Dehumanization of Man* [1970] (Syracuse: Syracuse University Press, 1991).

Szasz, T., *Insanity: The Idea and Its Consequences* [1987] (Syracuse: Syracuse University Press, 1997).

Szasz, T., *A Lexicon of Lunacy: Metaphoric Malady, Moral Responsibility, and Psychiatry* (New Brunswick, NJ: Transaction Publishers, 1993).

Szasz, T., *The Manufacture of Madness: A Comparative Study of the Inquisition and the Mental Health Movement* [1970] (Syracuse: Syracuse University Press, 1997).

Szasz, T., *The Meaning of Mind: Language, Morality, and Neuroscience* [1996] (Syracuse: Syracuse University Press, 2002).

Szasz, T., *The Myth of Mental Illness: Foundations of a Theory of Personal Conduct* [1961]. Revised edition (New York: HarperCollins, 1974).

Szasz, T., *The Myth of Psychotherapy: Mental Healing as Religion, Rhetoric, and Repression* [1978] (Syracuse: Syracuse University Press, 1988).

Szasz, T., *Pharmacracy: Medicine and Politics in America* [2001] (Syracuse: Syracuse University Press, 2003).

Szasz, T., *Schizophrenia: The Sacred Symbol of Psychiatry* [1976] (Syracuse: Syracuse University Press, 1988).

Szasz, T., *The Therapeutic State: Psychiatry in the Mirror of Current Events* (Buffalo: Prometheus Books, 1984).

Szasz, T., editor, *The Age of Madness: A History of Involuntary Mental Hospitalization Presented in Selected Texts* (Garden City, N.Y.: Doubleday Anchor, 1973).

Trombley, S., *All That Summer She Was Mad: Virginia Woolf, Female Victim of Male Medicine* (New York: Continuum, 1981).

Ussher, J. M., *Women's Madness: Misogyny or Mental Illness?* (Amherst: University of Massachusetts Press, 1991).

Woodward, K. L., *Making Saints: How the Catholic Church Determines Who Becomes a Saint, Who Doesn't, and Why* (New York: Simon and Schuster, 1990).

Woolf, L., *Beginning Again: An Autobiography of the Years 1911-1918* (New York: Harcourt, Brace & World, 1964).

Woolf, L., *The Journey Not the Arrival Matters: An Autobiography of the Years 1939-1969* (New York: Harcourt Brace Jovanovich, 1969).

Woolf, L., *The Letters of Leonard Woolf*. Edited by Frederic Spotts (Harcourt Brace Jovanovich, 1989).

Woolf, L. and Strachey, J., editors, *Virginia Woolf and Lytton Strachey: Letters* (New York: Harcourt, Brace & Co., 1956).

Woolf, V., *The Diary of Virginia Woolf, Volumes I-III, 1915-1930*. Edited by Anne Olivier Bell (New York: Harcourt Brace Jovanovich, 1977-80).

Woolf, V., *The Letters of Virginia Woolf*. Edited by Nigel Nicolson and Joanne Trautmann (6 vols.; New York: Harcourt Brace Jovanovich, 1975-80).

Woolf, V., *Moments of Being: Unpublished Autobiographical Writings*. Edited by Jeanne Schulkind (London: Sussex University Press, 1976).

Woolf, V., *Mrs. Dalloway* [1925] (New York: Harcourt Brace & World, 1935).

Woolf, V., *On Being Ill* (London: Hogarth Press, 1930).

Woolf, V., *A Room of One's Own* [1929] (New York: Harvest Books, 1989).

Woolf, V., *A Writer's Diary: Being Extracts from the Diary of Virginia Woolf*. Edited by Leonard Woolf (New York: Signet/New American Library, 1968).

Zweig, S., *Mental Healers: Franz Anton Mesmer, Mary Baker Eddy, Sigmund Freud* [1931]. Translated by Eden and Cedar Paul (New York: Frederick Ungar, 1962).

Zwerdling, Alex, *Virginia Woolf and the Real World* (Berkeley: University of California Press, 1986).

Acknowledgments

Once again, I wish to acknowledge my gratitude to Peter Uva and his colleagues at the library of the Upstate Medical University of the State University of New York in Syracuse for their generous and devoted help.

I thank Elizabeth Daly for her careful reading of the manuscript and useful suggestions; Mira de Vries, Keith Hoeller, Alice Michtom, Jeffrey Schaler, and Roger Yanow for critiquing the manuscript; Anthony and Naomi Stadlen for their encouragement and counsel; Michael Paley, my editor at Transaction Publishers, for his conscientious preparation of the text for publication; and my brother George, daughters Margot Peters and Susan Palmer, and son-in-law Steve Peters for their loving advice.

Index